A Cardiologist's Guide to . . .

Anti-Aging, Antioxidants & Resveratrol

A Cardiologist's Guide to . . .

Anti-Aging, Antioxidants & Resveratrol

How Red Wine Extract, Resveratrol and Super Antioxidants are Conquering

Heart Disease • Cancer • Diabetes
Alzheimer's • Obesity • Old Age

Dr. William S. Gruss, M.D.

Renaissance Health Education, LLC
Boca Raton, Florida

Published by
Renaissance Health Education, LLC
925 S. Federal Highway, Suite 500
Boca Raton, Florida 33432
www.naturalhealthnewsreport.com

Printed in the United States of America

ISBN 0-9800855-0-0

10   9   8   7   6   5   4   3   2   1

This book is designed to provide information about good health. It is sold with the understanding that the publisher is not engaged in rendering professional services. If medical treatment is required, please contact a doctor or other health professional.

CONTENTS

ACKNOWLEDGMENTS

I want to acknowledge the individuals who paved the way for me to write this book—the result of my exploration into a new realm of medical science. First, I give infinite love and thanks to my beautiful wife, Laurie, and to my two fantastic daughters, Jillian (15), and Gina Marie (8), for their unending support, love, and understanding. Having a busy medical practice, researching and writing this book, plus all the demands of *life* squeezed my time with them from every angle. They were incredibly patient.

I also want to thank my close friend, James DiGeorgia, owner of Renaissance Health, who asked me to investigate a product that he wanted to develop and market. He thought my background would make me a natural choice as an investigator and doctor spokesperson. This investigation into the health benefits of a product that included resveratrol found in red wine, red wine extract, and the other antioxidants I discuss in this book, gave me the opportunity to expand an enjoyable hobby—red wine—into my practice of medicine. The practice of medicine was becoming progressively frustrating (that's the subject for another book), and I was hungry for a different kind of knowledge.

I had the great fortune to work on this book with Mairi Ross. She has been tireless in helping me review, retrieve, and reclassify all the materials, including the scientific studies listed as sources. She has also interviewed me to elicit and clarify my thoughts. This was critical in helping me organize all the information for this book.

There is growing support for a new perspective in medicine. My office staff has been supportive from the beginning, promoting the alternative health solutions found in this book to friends and patients who showed an interest. I have been amazed how receptive my patients, relatives and friends have been. Many are now taking red wine extract, resveratrol, acetyl L-carnitine, alpha lipoic acid, and quercetin.

Little did I know that serving a double-magnum bottle of a vintage 1988 red wine—Brunello di Montalcino—at my engagement party over 12 years ago would lead to a new health product, a tremendous amount of new knowledge, and this book. In Italian, they toast with an expression, "A hundred years!" Let us make it a hundred healthy years and beyond!

William S. Gruss, M.D.

INTRODUCTION
A CARDIOLOGIST'S
JOURNEY—FROM HEART
ATTACKS TO
ANTIOXIDANTS

I was educated as a conventional medical doctor specializing in cardiology and internal medicine. After finishing medical school at the University of Maryland in 1981, I moved to South Florida and did my internal medicine residency and cardiology fellowship at Mount Sinai Hospital in Miami Beach. Part of my training was also at the University of Miami's Jackson Memorial Hospital. I spent five years in Miami and in 1986 started my private practice in Boca Raton, Florida, where I still practice today.

I have seen many changes in cardiology, both in the attitude of doctors and the technical practice of medicine during the last 26 years. When I was in my internship and residency there was a great deal of pessimism about aging and heart disease. I observed patients in their mid-60s coming in with heart attacks and other heart problems. At the time, they'd be scheduled for cardiac catheterization, bypass surgery, or other procedures. At the start of my training years in 1981, some senior attending physicians were very negative about these patients. They would say, "He's 65 years old. He's old. Why are we doing all these procedures on him?" The doctors just didn't think there was any use doing these procedures on such "old" people.

As time went on, technology improved and patients even older than 65 were able to survive these procedures and continue to live with a reasonably good quality of life. The latest research by Dr. Keith A. Fox, professor of cardiology at the University of Edinburgh in Scotland and published in the May, 2007, issue of the *Journal of the American Medical Association (JAMA)* shows that aggressive use of angioplasty and current heart medications have dramatically improved the survival rate for acute heart events like heart failure and heart attacks. Heart medications have improved and become more convenient for patients, increasing compliance. They can now be taken only once a day instead of four times a day and the side effects have been reduced.

Now, due to improved procedures and medication, people are getting older and older and two things are happening. The first thing is that younger people are looking at people having all these procedures and they think, "Oh my God, I don't want to have a heart attack. I don't want to have a stroke and go through all of that." These people start wanting to reduce their risk factors. They start researching and finding out how to do that. They stop smoking, improve their diet, avoid trans fats, reduce salt, and exercise regularly. They research on the Internet and they read about supplements and they take them as well. The second thing is that older people who have survived these procedures want to feel better. They don't want to just survive, they want to have energy and a good quality of life. They, too, start to read and gather information and many of them start taking supplements.

I discovered some of this when I asked my patients what medicine they take. My patients would tell me, "Oh, I have my blood pressure pill and my cholesterol pill." And that would be all they were taking. Then I'd ask, "Are you taking any supplements?" It just amazed me how many supplements everyone was taking. People really are looking for alternatives to medication and medical procedures. They're tired of the side effects and some patients are very concerned about the high cost as well.

Since my patients were looking for alternatives, I started reading and doing research as well. Then, about three years ago, I was asked to review a combination of antioxidant supplements that included resveratrol from red wine, alpha lipoic acid, acetyl L-carnitine, quercetin, and a red wine and grape seed extract that contained a high level (95%) of oligomeric proanthocyanidins (OPCs). In order to accurately review this product, I had to dig deeper and learn more about this new world of antioxidant supplements for heart health and anti-aging.

Of course, I was skeptical. I had never opposed my patients taking supplements, but I'd usually say something like, "Oh, they probably won't harm you" or "Well, at least you'll have a healthy toilet," implying that most of the properties of the supplement would pass through them into the toilet.

As I researched these five supplements, however, I was amazed at what I found. One of the first things I ran across was what is called the French Paradox. In France they eat a lot of rich, creamy foods and many of the people are heavy smokers, yet they don't have the level of coronary disease you would expect to see. Their rate of heart disease is much lower than the U.S. It seemed that the answer to the French Paradox was in the red wine. Something in the red wine gave them added protection. I discovered that red wine has high concentrations of resveratrol, an extraordinary compound with anti-aging, anticancer, and antioxidant benefits. Plus it contains OPCs that are also powerful antioxidants, quercetin that is a strong anti-inflammatory, and several other beneficial compounds as well. The benefits from these antioxidants were impressive. I discovered that these red wine antioxidants maintain a healthy level of nitric oxide in the body that helps prevent heart disease. This medical discovery won the Nobel Prize, yet many cardiologists are still unaware of it.

I became more and more intrigued by the research I was reading. There were quite a few animal studies, some small human studies, and some large population studies that focused on diet and red wine and health. The results of the studies of red wine showed that it seemed to be the magic factor. There have been attempts to negate that, but it's been shown consistently that people who drink red wine with high levels of OPCs and resveratrol and who eat fruits and vegetables have dramatically lower rates of heart disease. So, even though I am a conventional medical doctor who prescribes medication, if there are other things that can be helpful, I ask, why not include that in what I'm doing?

I also happen to be someone who enjoys a glass of red wine. My parents, born in Buenos Aires, Argentina, immigrated to the United States in 1952. Argentina is the fifth largest red wine producing country. I grew up appreciating how adults would enjoy a glass of red wine with meals. Now, I don't drink it every night, but certainly I enjoy it socially and occasionally at home. I like to read about different types of red wine and have become knowledgeable and educated about it. When I started to realize that red wine had some medical benefits, especially for the heart, I wanted to learn more about it.

I discovered that antioxidants that come from red wine have great benefits in helping to reduce the risk of heart disease. Because antioxidants prevent the oxidation of bad cholesterol (LDL) they help prevent plaque formation that leads to atherosclerosis. Antioxidants also prevent the oxidation of good cholesterol (HDL) so that the good cholesterol can sweep up the bad cholesterol and do a better job in keeping the arteries healthy. Research is now indicating that resveratrol, one of the red wine antioxidants, may have profound neurological, anti-cancer, and anti-aging benefits as well.

Cardiologists used to think that heart health was all about cholesterol and blood pressure. Now, of course, research is showing that inflammation and oxidation are the two root causes of heart disease and other chronic diseases. In addition, the Nobel Prize-winning research on nitric oxide has revealed that the components in red wine help maintain healthy levels of this molecule. You may have heard how nitric oxide helps male erectile dysfunction. It's because of its effect on the vascular system, which also includes the heart. We are now realizing that nitric oxide is critical to the functioning of the mitochondria in every cell in the body. In this book, I'm going to tell you a lot about the mitochondria, which is the power center for every cell. Some scientists are calling this the age of "mitochondrial medicine" saying that "all roads lead to the mitochondria." I agree with them. All of the supplements in this book help keep the mitochondria healthy.

I also researched the super antioxidant alpha lipoic acid and its team member, acetyl L-carnitine, that work in the mitochondria. Dr. Bruce Ames at the University of California, Berkeley, has done some exciting research with these two supplements showing profound improvements in energy in aging rats. There has also been some recent human research using acetyl L-carnitine in cancer survivors to combat fatigue and increase energy. Mitochondria produce almost all your energy, so if you keep the mitochondria healthy, you're going to improve energy function.

As I researched further, I also found that antioxidant compounds promote the natural destruction of cancer cells, a process called apoptosis that happens in the mitochondria. They inhibit other mechanisms of cancer as well. People are afraid to even think about cancer. They are very fatalistic about it. I think that's because they don't know that they can take preventive measures. Taking antioxidant and anti-inflammatory supplements that protect the mitochondria of our cells may be able to reduce our risk of cancer significantly.

What I've realized is that people want to find every possible advantage so that they can enjoy life as long as possible. The longevity curve has been somewhat flat for the last 150 years. A man who reached 70 in 1850 could only expect to live to 79. A man reaching 70 in the year 2000 could expect to live to 82. There's not that much difference. However, I think we are going to see that curve start sloping up. People who are approaching 70 who have not been smoking, who watch what they eat, take mitochondrial antioxidants, exercise, and have a positive outlook on life are going to be hitting 70 running as opposed to just surviving. When people get to this age, they want to be in the best possible shape so they don't have to have the invasive medical procedures. Once you start surviving heart attacks, angioplasties, coronary bypasses, and carotid surgeries, it takes a lot out of you.

Heart disease is the number one killer in America. And even if you survive, it is very debilitating. It is the most sudden, lethal disease we have. So, in the back of everyone's mind is, how can I prevent this from happening to me? More and more of my patients are interested in primary prevention. They aren't having any symptoms, and they don't want to develop them. This is a big change. People are thinking ahead and doing something to prevent the problem from happening, and one of the things they are doing is taking supplements that are going to reduce inflammation and oxidation and increase nitric oxide—and that's going to make a huge difference.

One of the most profound insights that has helped me in preventive medicine is understanding that all chronic illness has two root causes: oxidation and inflammation. We tend to think that there is one cause for diabetes, another for heart disease, another for cancer. However, all chronic diseases have two things in common: oxidation and inflammation that damage cells, tissues and organs. The five supplements discussed in this book address these two root causes.

Once I realized this, I became committed to an anti-aging health program that includes these five supplements. I take resveratrol, quercetin, red wine extract containing 95% OPCs, alpha lipoic acid and acetyl L-carnitine. I take a mitochondrial multivitamin. I don't smoke. I try to eat well, exercise, reduce my salt intake, and lower my stress levels. There are some people who, genetically, are going to have high blood pressure and cholesterol and they'll have to take the medications. But it's possible to reduce your risk of heart disease very significantly by doing primary prevention prior to taking medication. I really think that these supplements can help people maintain their health for a much longer period of time. People have to realize that most of them will not feel something dramatic at first. For many people, the perceivable effects are subtle. However, others will notice more energy, less fatigue, and possibly a better sex life fairly soon.

When I started taking these supplements, most importantly, I felt no ill side effects. I noticed I had more energy, my blood sugar stabilized so I wasn't as hungry, I lost some weight, and my circulation improved. But the real payoff is going to be in the long-term effects of living a longer, healthier life.

I think our average life expectancy and quality of life is going to increase dramatically for a certain segment of the population that takes these preventive measures. These people are going to hit 70 with peak energy and vitality and keep going through their 90s and even get to 100 with a good quality of life. They won't be crippled and debilitated. I'm already starting to see this in my practice. In the last few years, I've started seeing more and more really older patients, mid to late 80s to mid 90s that are doing well. They come in to see me and they're still quite sharp. They're joking, they're getting around, some of them are still driving, and they are still enjoying life. That's the key. You want to live longer and still be able to enjoy life.

After years of research on these supplements, I wanted to share what I have learned so that you will have the opportunity to live into *your* later years with health and vitality. Resveratrol, quercetin, red wine extract with 95% OPCs, acetyl L-carnitine, and alpha lipoic acid may seem like long, complicated names to you right now. However, after you read this book, I believe you will get to know them and adopt them as trusted members of your personal wellness and anti-aging team.

Wishing you the best of health,

William S. Gruss, M.D.
Boca Raton, Florida

1
HEART DISEASE, RED WINE, AND THE FRENCH PARADOX

Having a heart attack is, justifiably, one of the worst fears of Americans as they age. A heart attack is sudden, painful, and often unexpected and lethal. About two-thirds of all unexpected cardiac deaths occur without the person even knowing they had a heart problem. Most Americans watch their cholesterol levels, but 50% of all heart attacks happen to people with "normal" cholesterol. Since 1900, heart disease has been the number one killer in the United States every year except 1918. Although many people think of heart disease as a men's problem, it is also the number one killer of women. One in three female deaths is from cancer, while 1 in 2.6 is from heart disease. Heart disease and cancer are the "Big Two," accounting for almost all disease mortality in the United States.[1]

Death from heart disease rises dramatically as you age. Deaths from heart disease and cancer are fairly equal until the age of 75 and then deaths from heart disease shoot up.[2] If you want to live longer and in better health, you must find a way to reduce your risk of heart disease. If you are *really* serious about living to 90 or 100 in good health, you will find a way to reduce your risk of heart disease *and* cancer.

Is it possible? Fortunately, as a practicing cardiologist, I can tell you the answer is a resounding yes! Research in the last 15 years has discovered new, natural, and safe ways to protect against heart disease, cancer, aging, and all chronic diseases. This book, based on the very latest discoveries, will tell you how.

EXPERTS WERE WRONG

Since the late 1950s, almost all cardiologists, the American Heart Association, governmental experts, and nutritionists have recommended to the American public that in order to prevent heart disease they must avoid red meat, cream, whole milk, cheese, butter, and eggs. They were told that foods that contain high levels of saturated fat and cholesterol would "clog their arteries." Americans were instructed in no uncertain terms that the way to reduce the risk of heart disease was to eat an overall low-fat, low-cholesterol diet. Tragically, the one fat that was recommended to be used instead of butter was margarine. We now know that margarine *increases* the risk of heart disease.[3]

The theory was that because the plaque in clogged arteries, a condition called atherosclerosis, contains high levels of cholesterol, lowering dietary cholesterol would prevent plaque and clogged arteries and reduce death from heart disease.[4] Unfortunately, it was not as simple as this.

FRENCH PARADOX SHOCKS AMERICA

Based on these recommendations, Americans and their doctors firmly believed that eating a low-fat, low-cholesterol diet was a sure path to avoiding a heart attack. That's why a report on the CBS television news show *60 Minutes* shocked the entire nation. This report, broadcast November 17, 1991, changed the direction of heart research and the prevention of heart disease in America and around the world.

Morley Safer, the host of the program, revealed that the French ate a lot of cheese, eggs, butter, and rich cream sauces, plus they smoked and didn't get much exercise, and they had up to a 40% *lower* death rate from heart disease than Americans. This is called the French Paradox. It was incredible. Americans had been told by the highest authorities that if they gave up their steaks and baked potatoes, their sour cream and butter, rich desserts, ice cream, and eggs and bacon with buttered toast it would protect them from heart attacks. Now, *60 Minutes*, a highly respected news program, was telling them that the French did all the things they weren't supposed to do and had less heart disease. How was this possible?

To answer this question, Safer interviewed two prestigious scientists: Dr. Serge Renaud from France and Dr. Curt Ellison, an American cardiologist and professor from the School of Public Health at Boston University. They both agreed that a moderate consumption of red wine might be the answer.[5] The French had the highest consumption of red wine in the world, and areas of France that drank the most red wine had the lowest levels of heart disease.[6] Could red wine be the magic elixir that protected the French from heart disease? How could red wine be healthy?

Wine experts recall the response to the show. "It had a major impact," said Ronn Wiegand, a well-known wine columnist. "At the time, neoprohibitionists were grouping wine with illegal drugs. Morale in the wine business was the lowest since I have been in the business and that's since 1972. Friends were leaving the business to get involved in something more acceptable."[7] Being told that drinking any kind of alcohol could be healthy was a completely new concept to most Americans. However, after the broadcast, sales of red wine increased 44% almost overnight.[8]

WAS THE FRENCH PARADOX TRUE?

Scientists scrambled to examine the research and conducted new research to find out if the French Paradox was true. Was drinking red wine really the answer to lowering deaths from heart attacks?[9] The implications were enormous. If the French Paradox could be transferred to America, and we could reduce deaths from heart disease by 40%, we would save tens of thousands of lives a year—without dangerous medications and operations—simply by drinking red wine!

Scientists scrutinized the data. Did the French really eat as much or more saturated fats as Americans and have up to 40% fewer deaths from heart disease? Did red wine help prevent death from heart disease? Was there something special about red wine and not other alcoholic drinks that prevented heart disease? If so, what was it? And, could you get the same effects if you isolated that something special and took away the alcohol?

Did the French eat high levels of saturated fat and have lower rates of heart disease?
Yes.

Although there have been numerous attempts in the years since 1991 to discount the French Paradox, none have succeeded. The first question asked by scientists was whether the cause of death in France due to heart disease was underestimated. Validated data on death due to heart disease show that the French do, in fact, have lower rates of death due to heart disease than other countries.[10] Surveys of the French population have shown their saturated fat intake is 15–16%, a level similar to Americans.[11]

Does drinking moderate amounts of red wine help prevent heart disease?
Yes.

Population studies indicate that within France red wine consumption is the highest in the south where deaths from heart disease are lowest. French people in the north consume more beer and spirits and they have a higher rate of death from heart disease.[12] Although studies show that moderate drinking of alcohol from any source has a protective effect against heart disease by raising HDL (good cholesterol), wine appears to have special benefits not found in other types of alcohol.[13]

Dr. Renaud, the French scientist interviewed on *60 Minutes*, published an important study in the prestigious medical journal *Lancet* in 1992 investigating the specific beneficial effects of red wine on the heart. He concluded that the specific benefit of red wine was not due to its effects on good cholesterol or the lowering of bad cholesterol. He found that cholesterol levels were about the same in France, the USA, and the United Kingdom. However, the mortality rates from heart disease were dramatically different: 78 deaths from heart disease per 100,000 people in Toulouse, France, compared to 182 in Stanford, California, USA, and 380 in Glasgow, Scotland.[14] The average number of deaths from heart attacks in the USA is 255 per 100,000, according to the American Heart Association (2004).

Next Dr. Renaud investigated the action of platelet aggregation, or the tendency of blood to clot and cause heart attacks. Aspirin, for example, is commonly used to reduce blood clotting and reduce deaths from heart attacks. He compared levels of platelet aggregation between farmers in Scotland and farmers in France. Farmers in France drank twice the amount of alcohol, primarily red wine, and they had strikingly lower platelet aggregation and lower numbers of deaths from heart disease. Renaud concluded that there was *something* in red wine that was protecting the blood from dangerous clots and preventing heart attacks.[15]

Another group of researchers found that red wine intake, but not another form of alcohol (vodka), prevented the activation of a component in the blood that causes lesions in the arteries. Lesions damage the arteries, cause inflammation and attract plaque that clogs arteries.[16] Other studies reported that the lowest risk of dying from heart disease was among those who drank red wine compared with those preferring other alcoholic beverages.[17] Since the television broadcast in 1991, several thousand studies have examined the connection between red wine and heart disease. A 2007 review of red wine research in the prestigious *European Heart Journal* concluded that red wine has a protective effect on the heart beyond the effect of the alcohol.[18]

What is it about red wine that's so special?
Resveratrol, OPCs, quercetin and other polyphenols.

Keeping all these names straight can be a challenge. All of the above compounds are in a group of natural plant chemicals called plant polyphenols. Flavonoids are also polyphenols, so you will also see some of these compounds referred to as flavonoids. Polyphenols includes all of them, so I'll refer to the group of healthy components in red wine as polyphenols. According to a leading cardiology researcher at State University in Buffalo, New York, "The unique cardioprotective properties of red wine reside in the action of polyphenol flavonoids, which are absent in white wine...." [19] Below are some of the leading candidates for the special "something" in red wine that results in the French Paradox. Because these polyphenols are so important to our health, I'll cover them in more detail in following chapters.

Resveratrol. Resveratrol, a nonflavonoid polyphenol, was the first compound that scientists investigated to explain the French Paradox. It is one of the most intriguing compounds found in nature. There are not many foods commonly eaten that have high levels of resveratrol. Resveratrol is produced in plants primarily in response to a stressor in the environment. In wine, it is commonly produced by the skin, leaves and canes of grape plants in response to a specific fungus. Because red wine is made with the skin of the grapes, it contains more resveratrol than white wine.

Because the presence of the stressor can vary depending on the weather, soil and other variables, not all red wine contains high levels of resveratrol. Levels of resveratrol in Pinot Noir may vary:[20]

Australia	13.4 mg/L
California	5.5 mg/L
Burgundy	4.4 mg/L
Spain	5.1 mg/L

It may be possible that therapeutic levels of resveratrol against heart disease could be reached by drinking wine.[21] This data could change, however. As herbicides and pesticides become more commonly used in grape cultivation, the level of resveratrol in red wine declines.

Another source of resveratrol is from the roots of the Japanese knotweed plant (*Polygonum cuspidatum*). Most commercial supplements will contain resveratrol from the knotweed plant as it is more consistent and easier to extract.

As the research on resveratrol exploded, there was more and more evidence that resveratrol had many cardioprotective properties. It protected arteries from the oxidation of bad cholesterol; suppressed inflammation that can damage arteries and cause the build up of plaque; reduced the tendency of the blood to clot and cause strokes and heart attacks; increased the release of nitric oxide which relaxes blood vessels and inhibits atherosclerosis; and helped prevent damage from heart attacks.[22] [23]

There have been thousands of studies on resveratrol, not only its cardioprotective properties, but anticancer, anti-aging, and insulin normalizing properties as well. There are still questions to be answered about the bioavailability of resveratrol and other antioxidants and how they work. I'll discuss antioxidants in more detail in Chapter 3 and new research on resveratrol in Chapter 6.

Resveratrol is truly one of the miracle molecules of nature, but is it the magic ingredient in red wine that prevents heart disease? Other components of red wine have also been investigated and found to benefit the heart.

OPCs and anthocyanidins. The next candidates to be investigated were flavonoid polyphenols called oligomeric proanthocyanidins (also called OPCs). Closely related but slightly different are procyanidins and anthocyanidins. OPCs are derived from grape seeds and anthocyanidins from grape skins.These are strong anti-oxidants and help support the health of arteries, veins and capillaries. Although resveratrol was the early contender for the title of the "magic ingredient" in red wine, OPCs and anthocyanidins have also been gaining recognition as potent cardioprotective compounds. I will discuss more about them in Chapter 8.

Quercetin. Quercetin is a powerful anti-inflammatory, antioxidant, and is also a flavonoid polyphenol. Quercetin is available from food sources such as onions, apples, grapes and other fruits and vegetables. Quercetin improves the absorption of resveratrol, as well as having its own positive effects on preventing heart diseases.[24][25] In a dietary study of over 100,000 persons for one year, those with a higher intake of quercetin had less coronary heart disease.[26] There are still other antioxidant flavonoids in red wine such as catechin that have been shown to help prevent heart disease.[27]

And the winner is...? Nature did not create each of the above compounds in isolation. In their natural state in red wine, they come together as a package. Perhaps it is no coincidence that red wine is one of the most chemically complex foods. It's very possible that the health benefits of red wine are a result of the interaction of all of the compounds in the whole grape, skin and seeds. Multiple mechanisms of benefit and action are very probable.[28]

The French Paradox started a landslide of research into all of the above compounds with some startling results. Scientists discovered that the above compounds from red wine not only protect our hearts, they also protect against cancer, diabetes, Alzheimer's, and all the chronic diseases of aging. Most importantly, they support our mitochondria, the source of life and death in all cells in our body. And one of the compounds may hold the key to extending human life. I will discuss all of these amazing benefits of red wine in the following chapters.

Can you get the same results without the alcohol? Yes.

Once the scientific community discovered that it could be resveratrol, quercetin, OPCs and other polyphenols in red wine responsible for its protective benefits, they investigated to find out whether these benefits existed without the alcohol. Scientists discovered that red wine, powdered red wine extract, dealcoholized red wine, and purple grape juice all act in the same way. You can get the benefits of red wine without the alcohol. I prefer a red wine extract that contains high (95%) levels of OPCs from grape seeds plus grape skin anthocyanins.

One excellent study concluded that taking an oral supplement of red wine extract lowered blood pressure in rats. The supplement produced a progressive decrease in systolic blood pressure within four days. The red wine supplement relaxed the arteries due to increased nitric oxide activity.[29] Other studies showed that red wine extract lowers oxidation and the blood clotting mechanism. Remember, oxidation is one of the two root causes of disease. It is not the level of cholesterol but the level of *oxidation of cholesterol* that is the critical factor in artery damage.[30][31][32][33][34][35] I will present much more information about oxidation in the coming chapters.

MAYBE IT WASN'T THE FAT AFTER ALL

One of the main premises of the French Paradox, however, may not be true. The underlying premise of the paradox is that all fat, but especially saturated fat and foods high in cholesterol, is a high risk factor for heart disease. As research has continued, more scientists are questioning whether natural dietary fats have any impact on heart disease. A review of all the best studies by the prestigious Cochrane Institute in 2001 found that reducing or modifying dietary fat had no effect on deaths from heart disease or deaths from any cause.[36] Another study published in the *Journal of the American Medical Association* found that lowering total fat in the diet is unlikely to improve cholesterol levels or reduce the incidence of heart disease.[37] The famous Framingham Study of a population in New York that has been used as a basis for heart research all over the world, stated that no relation was found between eating foods high in saturated fat and cholesterol and blood cholesterol levels.[38] A study of over 43,000 male health professionals found that intake of total fat, cholesterol, high-fat dairy products, nuts, and eggs were not related to risk of stroke.[39]

The largest, most expensive study ever conducted to discover whether a low-fat diet reduces the risk of heart disease and cancer came up with a convincing no! The Harvard School of Public Health online newsletter states that this study proved a low-fat diet does not prevent heart disease or cancer and does not help people lose weight, either. The study followed 50,000 women between the ages of 50 and 79 who were assigned to either follow a low-fat diet or to continue their usual diets. This study cost hundreds of millions of dollars and lasted eight years. *The New York Times* quoted Dr. Michael Thun who directs research for the American Cancer Society, "This was the Rolls-Royce of studies. It is likely to be the final word because we usually have only one shot at a very large-scale trial on a particular issue."[40] The results, the study investigators agreed, do not justify recommending low-fat diets to the public to reduce their heart disease and cancer risk.

The study was published in the February, 2006, *Journal of the American Medical Association,* and showed no benefits for a low-fat diet. It did not protect against heart disease, breast cancer, colorectal cancer, or keep weight down.[41]

In contrast to these human trials, some laboratory and mouse studies do show that high calorie diets that contain a very high amount of fat (60%) increase oxidation and inflammation and lead to heart disease, diabetes, and other indicators of age and illness.[42] Common sense and research tell us that eating healthy fats such as olive oil and nuts in a diet rich in fruits, vegetables, and whole grains and a moderate amount of saturated fat from grass-fed, high omega-3 animals is healthy. Eating a diet high in French fries, pastries, cookies, margarine, lunch meats, hot dogs, and other unhealthy fatty foods is…unhealthy.

THERE IS ONE KIND OF VERY BAD FAT

The only type of fat that *has* been found to be clearly associated with heart disease is trans fat. Margarine and other partially hydrogenated oils found in almost all commercial pastries, cookies, crackers, pancakes, and breads and other processed foods are trans fats. Tragically, margarine was recommended as a heart-healthy fat for many years. Now we know that it causes inflammation and raises the oxidation of LDL cholesterol, damaging arteries. Harvard researchers have found that eliminating trans fats from the food supply could prevent tens of thousands of heart attacks and deaths from heart disease every year.[43]

Some researchers even suspect that the epidemic of heart disease has been caused by trans fats.

IF NOT FAT, THEN WHAT'S CAUSING DEATHS FROM HEART DISEASE?

If eating a low-fat, low-cholesterol diet doesn't reduce our risk for heart disease, what does? It's crucial to be able to identify accurately the risks for heart disease, cancer and other chronic diseases so that people can take action to reduce those risks and thereby reduce their risk of illness. In the next chapter, I will review what public health authorities now advise are the highest risks for chronic illness and tell you why I think they've missed the two root causes of all chronic diseases. Then I'll tell you how red wine extract, resveratrol, quercetin, alpha lipoic acid, and acetyl L-carnitine can address the two root causes of all chronic diseases—oxidation and inflammation. They can help reduce your risk of heart disease and all chronic diseases of aging—even aging itself!

2
THE CRUSHING BURDEN OF CHRONIC DISEASE IN AMERICA—CANCER, HEART DISEASE, DIABETES, AND ALZHEIMER'S

The United States spends more money per person on health care than any other country in the world, yet it ranks only 42nd in life expectancy. Countries that surpass the United States include Japan, most of Europe, Jordan, Guam and the Cayman Islands. The United States is not keeping up. Twenty years ago, it ranked 11th. "Something's wrong here when one of the richest countries in the world, the one that spends the most on health care, is not able to keep up with other countries," said Dr. Christopher Murray, head of the Institute for Health Metrics and Evaluation at the University of Washington, in an Associated Press story, August 11, 2007.[1]

This is not news to health professionals in America. The burden of chronic disease is growing heavier and heavier, crushing 85% of all seniors with at least one chronic illness. Forty-five percent of the working population has a chronic illness, which is defined as a condition that lasts a year or more and requires ongoing medical attention and/or limits activities of daily living. Four out of five health care dollars are spent on people with chronic conditions. The authors of this shocking report on chronic disease say these numbers *underestimate* the problem.[2] In human terms, chronic illness means it's hard for you to get up without pain, to go to work, walk easily, to shop and cook, to play with your grandchildren without being out of breath, or to have the energy to get together with friends and family. It means you spend a lot of your time and money in doctors' offices or hospitals and paying for prescription medications instead of getting ahead in your career, buying a new car, golfing, gardening, dancing, or traveling with loved ones.

The most common chronic illnesses are heart disease, high blood pressure, arthritis, diabetes, eye disorders and chronic mental conditions like Alzheimer's. Although not listed as a chronic disease, cancer takes a daily toll on the people who are fighting it. I consider it a chronic disease. Every year, cancer is diagnosed in more than a million people, and half a million die from it—that means many people are living with it. Having more than one condition is common. For example, 70% of people with high blood pressure have at least one other chronic condition.[3]

Although Americans have one of the highest standards of living in the world, we pay for it in an environment that has high levels of indoor and outdoor pollution, noise, crime, and stress. We have a fast-paced life and a culture based on advertising that encourages eating from fast-food chains and restaurants where it's hard to get economical, nutritious meals.

High cholesterol, high blood pressure, high levels of blood sugar in diabetes, high levels of pain in arthritis, high stress, high cortisol, a high number of people with obesity—this is the landscape of chronic illness. Plus, the aging of our population raises the risk of chronic illness. Though the highest percentage of people who are ill are seniors, the greatest number of people with chronic illnesses are now of working age and privately insured—their chronic illnesses will only get worse as they age. Prescription medications for heart disease, diabetes, arthritis and other chronic illnesses can "manage" the symptoms of these diseases, but medicine can't prevent or cure them.

What is going on here in America? Our entire society is burdened with illness. The big question, of course, is can anything be done about it? I have written this book to tell you that something *can* be done about it. Scientific breakthroughs like the ones I will be telling you about in this book—resveratrol, alpha lipoic acid, acetyl L-carnitine, quercetin, and red wine polyphenols that go to the root causes of chronic diseases—are revealing the real possibility of a healthy aging population—not just old, but old and energetic and living life to the fullest.

HEART DISEASE DECLINES—WHY?

The good news is that deaths from heart disease are declining. Although heart disease is still the biggest killer, the rate of death has fallen 50% between 1980 and 2000.[4]

Of course, what people want to know is what is causing this decline in deaths from heart disease, so we can do more of it! The answer is, we really don't know for sure. Some experts suggest that it is better medical procedures and medications. The latest research indicates that about half the reduction is due to positive life- style changes and the other half to advances in medical care. Decreases in smoking, cholesterol, blood pressure and more exercise are the main lifestyle changes thought to reduce deaths.[5]

However, there may be other reasons for this decline

that are less obvious to the medical establishment. For example, we learned in the first chapter that drinking red wine high in the polyphenol antioxidants resveratrol, quercetin, and OPCs reduces your chance of getting heart disease by almost 40%.

A Yale School of Medicine researcher, Bauer Sumpio, M.D., professor and section chief of vascular surgery in the Department of Surgery, says that his laboratory found that it's red wine polyphenols that prevent plaque on the smooth muscle cells of arteries, inhibit platelet formation which can lead to blood clotting, and slow cell deterioration. A better understanding of the health benefits of red wine and the specific polyphenolic extracts would be a great contribution to society," Sumpio said.[6]

Wine consumption has doubled in the United States since the 1970s, and almost half of wine drinkers drink red wine.[7] It's absolutely possible that the increase in adults drinking red wine high in the polyphenols resveratrol, quercetin, and OPCs plus the consumption of dietary supplements with these and other antioxidants, may be contributing to the reduction in heart disease, cancer and other chronic diseases. I agree with Dr. Sumpio that educating the public about the benefits of these red wine polyphenols would be a great service and could reduce deaths from heart disease.

WHAT DO THE EXPERTS SAY WILL REDUCE YOUR RISK OF HEART DISEASE, CANCER, DIABETES, AND OTHER CHRONIC DISEASES?

It's important to understand the conventional recommendations and advice about chronic illness. This chapter will examine the standard risks for these diseases and what the authorities say to do about them. If you are interested in not only living a long life, but a healthy one, then it's important to know the risk factors for the most prevalent chronic diseases. A risk factor is something that increases your chance of having the problem. Once you know the risk factors, you can take steps to reduce them and prevent these conditions from making you a statistic.

However, we will also take a very close look at what the authorities could be missing and what alternative solutions may give you an even greater opportunity to reduce your risk of cancer and chronic illness. If the authorities get it wrong, millions of people will be doing what they think will reduce their risk, when it really doesn't. This is what has happened with the recommendations to eat a low-fat, low-cholesterol diet. By focusing on eating low fat and cutting out foods with cholesterol, people thought they were reducing their risk of heart disease, but they really weren't. If health authorities are looking in the wrong direction, they can overlook an important solution—like the ingredients in red wine—which is what I believe has happened. Doctors and nutritionists have been too focused on what *not* to eat (when it has turned out it didn't matter), and failed to focus on what *to* drink and eat that can make a difference.

One of the biggest and most damaging errors made by the authorities in the last 50 years was in recommending that people prevent heart disease by eating margarine full of dangerous trans fats. We now know that trans fats significantly *increase* heart disease and many other diseases by increasing oxidation of fats and inflammation in arteries. Trans fats are so dangerous that a government spokesman has declared there's no safe level. Denmark has banned trans fats and so has New York City. I hope many other cities will follow.

Combined Risk Factors for Heart Disease, Diabetes, High Blood Pressure, Arthritis, and Cancer That Can Be Modified[8]

- Smoking or environmental smoke
- Obesity
- Not exercising
- High stress
- Diet low in fruits and vegetables
- Diet high in all types of fat
- Diet high in saturated fat and cholesterol
- Diet high in sugar
- Diet high in trans fats
- High levels of salt
- Diabetes
- High cholesterol or abnormal blood lipids
- High blood pressure

Combined Recommended Solutions

- Stop smoking
- Exercise daily for 30 minutes
- Lose weight
- Lower stress
- Eat a low-fat, low-cholesterol diet
- Eat vegetables and fruits (5–10 servings a day)
- Control diabetes
- Manage cholesterol and blood pressure
- If you drink, drink in moderation (one drink a day for women, two a day for men)

WHAT DID THEY MISS?

Reducing the risk of clotting or platelet aggregation can reduce risk of a heart attack. Currently, most cardiologists prescribe a daily aspirin to achieve this reduction. Dr. Renaud's research on red wine suggested that it was the decreased platelet aggregation or blood clotting by red wine that lowered the risk of heart disease.[9] There have been a number of studies showing resveratrol's ability to reduce platelet aggregation.[10] A small 2006 study on high-risk cardiac patients who were resistant to aspirin showed that resveratrol effectively inhibited platelet aggregation. And resveratrol doesn't cause bleeding like aspirin does.[11] Today, fifty million people take aspirin to reduce blood clotting even though all conventional doses of aspirin are associated with gastrointestinal bleeding.[12] Taking aspirin may help reduce the risk of cardiovascular disease, but it also has significant side effects.

WHAT *ELSE* DID THEY MISS?

Although I agree with many of the risks listed, the experts missed the opportunity to *identify the two root causes of every chronic disease—inflammation and oxidation*. That's a lot to miss. They listed the symptoms, but not the cause. When you know the root causes of disease, you can find better specific solutions for preventing disease. It's not enough to advise you to "manage your cholesterol and blood pressure." You need to know how to do that. In the next chapter I will show you that each and every risk factor named by the authorities has these two root causes that are related to each other. By knowing what the root causes are, you can then start doing something about them.

LOOKING FOR ALTERNATIVES

Although I practice conventional medicine, I know that surgeries and prescription medications cannot cure or prevent heart disease, diabetes, cancer and other chronic illnesses. And I know that the practice of medicine has no answer for aging. My own research has convinced me that there *are* alternatives that can help people prevent chronic diseases and even aging. In order to write this book, I have reviewed hundreds of research studies that support this. Natural supplements like resveratrol, alpha lipoic acid, acetyl L-carnitine, red wine extract, and quercetin can make a difference in your quality of life—and may even extend the number of years you live.

That the standard solutions aren't working for many people is evident in their desire to find alternatives. My patients are hungry for good information that will help them be healthy—without the debilitating side effects of medications. The Internet has opened up a gold mine of information about natural solutions and supplements that don't cause dangerous side effects or cost a fortune. By some estimates, 40–50% of Americans now take a dietary supplement. Many of these people are on limited incomes and wouldn't be spending the money if they didn't feel they were getting a benefit.

That's why this book examines the real evidence about risk factors for chronic diseases, cancer and aging. The American people cannot afford another health disaster like trans fats. Unfortunately, many effective natural or alternative solutions are being ignored or falsely criti-cized—even if the scientific evidence shows that these solutions may be the key to preventing illness and disability. Many risk factors such as trans fats, sodas, and other junk foods are underpublicized due to powerful economic interests. You will notice in the list of solutions recommended by the health authorities, there is no mention of using supplements to lower inflammation and oxidation— the two root causes of all chronic illness. In the following chapters I will share with you the results of my research about natural, safe solutions that will help you stay healthy as you age.

3
TWO ROOT CAUSES OF ALL CHRONIC DISEASES— INFLAMMATION AND OXIDATION

Aging, chronic diseases and cancer are *all* associated with increased inflammation and oxidation. *All* of the valid risk factors for chronic diseases increase oxidation or inflammation or both. The two are connected. They are the root causes of disease and aging. As Dr. Andrew Weil, M.D. said on his Web site, "Chronic inflammation just may be the root of all degenerative diseases." A special report in the cancer medical journal *Oncology* concurred with Dr. Weil. "A substantial body of evidence supports the conclusion that chronic inflammation can predispose individuals to cancer... the longer the inflammation persists, the higher the risk."[1] If we can reduce chronic inflammation and oxidation, we can improve the prevention of every chronic disease—even cancer and aging. I believe we can do it.

WHAT IS INFLAMMATION?

Inflammation is nature's way of telling us that something is going wrong in our body. Inflammation is our basic defense and all inflammation begins with a triggering event. A bacteria, virus, parasite or toxin invades the body; a blow, fall, or surgery injures the body; or you eat food that is harmful and it sets off your alarm sentinels. After the inflammatory trigger has been pulled, white blood cells (macrophages) rush to the area where the invader has entered or the injury has occurred and free radicals increase.[2]

Macrophages produce proinflammatory cytokines, chemical messengers that attack and clean up cells in the affected area. If the inflammatory trigger continues, cytokine production rises, sending more and more signals to destroy more and more cells, and more and more free radicals are produced, which eventually leads to tissue and organ damage. For example, if you have continual inflammation in your knee, macrophages and free radicals will continue to attack the cartilage, destroying it, until you have none left.[3]

WHAT ARE FREE RADICALS AND OXIDATIVE STRESS?

When we breathe oxygen, the process of turning oxygen into energy in our cells creates free radicals. Free radicals (also called ROS or RONS) are molecules that want to grab electrons from other molecules. When a molecule loses an electron, that is called oxidation. It's kind of like a troublesome bachelor at a party trying to grab other men's dates.[4] By snatching electrons, free radicals can damage all types of cells in the body, including their DNA. In addition to energy production, other natural processes such as fighting infections and inflammation can create free radicals.

Antioxidants are molecules that give free radicals an

electron so they won't continue to cause problems. When the antioxidants can't keep up with the free radicals, it's called oxidative stress.

In addition to the normal production of free radicals and oxidized cells by the body's own mechanisms of breathing and inflammation, outside influences can also trigger the production of free radicals and oxidation. Environmental pollutants, cigarette smoke, radiation, ultraviolet light, drugs, medicines, pesticides, solvents, house cleaning toxins, weed killers, ozone, stress, trans fats, high levels of sugar, obesity and intense exercise all either create inflammation, which triggers oxidation, or trigger oxidation directly. You can see from the list that many of these outside triggers of inflammation and oxidation are due to our modern lifestyle.

HOW DO WE STOP FREE RADICAL DAMAGE?

If nature creates a problem, then nature usually creates a solution.

Our body produces powerful antioxidant enzymes to balance the normal oxidation process inside the cell. Some of the most important antioxidant enzymes are superoxide dismutase (SOD), catalase, and glutathione peroxidase. These enzymes reduce the concentrations of the most harmful oxidants. What's really important is that in order for our body to create these enzymes, it must have the minerals selenium, copper, manganese and zinc from food or supplements to create them. If you are deficient in any of these micronutrients—and many Americans are—you will not be able to make enough antioxidant enzymes to control free radicals.

But that's not all. Nature also created powerful antioxidants within our bodies. An antioxidant is a special kind of molecule that is stable enough to voluntarily give a rampaging free radical an extra electron so it will just settle down and stop grabbing electrons. Your body produces its own antioxidants such as alpha lipoic acid, nitric oxide, glutathione, ubiquinol (coenzyme Q-10), and uric acid.

However, our internal team needs reinforcement antioxidants, especially when the rate of oxidation is high. The modern lifestyle that includes high stress, toxins, pollutants, smoke, trans fats and sugar increases the need for outside antioxidant reinforcements.[5] Those reinforcements traditionally came from a diet very high in freshly picked fruits, vegetables and herbs plus drinks like red wine, tea, cocoa, and coffee.

If the body gets overwhelmed with too much oxidation and damage to cells, and does not have enough nutrients, enzymes and antioxidants to protect it, the oxidation damage gets ahead of the repair system and causes chronic inflammation, disease and aging. That's The Free Radical Theory of Aging.[6] I'll tell you in Chapter 9 why it's simply not possible to get all the antioxidant power you need from food.

AGING, CHRONIC INFLAMMATION AND FREE RADICALS

In some cases, especially in the elderly, the body loses its ability to down-regulate inflammation. It is normal for your body to respond with inflammation when there is a triggering event. Inflammation goes up, and once the danger has been averted, it goes back down. That's normal. When it doesn't go back down—that's trouble.[7]

Scientists are looking closely at the relationship of chronic inflammation and aging. They have discovered that chronic inflammation as we age impairs the ability of cells to get rid of damaging free radicals. Young organisms can down-regulate both inflammation and oxidation better than old organisms.[8] If inflammation and oxidation continue, then the free radicals continue to generate a cascade of chemicals that damage the cell, the tissue and eventually the organ. Once the organ sustains a significant amount of damage, the deterioration of health begins that results in chronic disease and aging.[9]

It's important to realize that it's normal to have inflammation and oxidation. Creating drugs that would completely suppress oxidation or inflammation would cause even more problems. A normal inflammation response protects you from infection and the process of oxidation helps kill off damaged cells that could lead to cancer.[10] However, inflammation and oxidative stress are now at "epidemic" levels and are out of control due to poor diet, toxic chemicals and stress. In order to reduce aging and chronic diseases you must reduce these two reactions in your body, especially as you age. Natural supplements like resveratrol, alpha lipoic acid, quercetin and red wine extract protect you against high levels of oxidation and inflammation without altering the natural balance within your body.

THE DISCOVERY OF CHRONIC INFLAMMATION AND ITS ROLE IN CHRONIC DISEASE

Just as the French Paradox stimulated the investigation into new ways to prevent heart disease, another paradox of heart disease started the research into chronic inflammation. As I noted in earlier chapters, up until the late 1990s, the medical community was committed to the concept that dietary fat and cholesterol clogged arteries with plaque and caused heart attacks. Anyone with high

Highly Sensitive C-Reactive Protein Test for Inflammation

Optimum Levels*

- Below 1.3 mg/L of blood is safe.
- Below 0.5 mg/L of blood is ideal.

*Even low levels of chronic inflammation can cause deterioration of tissue and lead to chronic diseases.

LDL cholesterol was told they were at great risk of having a heart attack.

There was only one problem—half of all heart attacks occurred in people with "normal" cholesterol levels. Plus, doctors found that the most dangerous plaques that built up in the arteries were not necessarily the large plaques and that they usually were not significantly blocking anything. Something else was causing the plaque deposits to burst, tear away from the artery wall and trigger massive clots that cut off the blood supply. In the early 1990s, Dr. Paul Ridker, a cardiologist at Brigham and Women's Hospital in Boston, became convinced that some sort of inflammatory reaction and not the build up of cholesterol was causing plaque to burst and cause heart attacks. He needed a simple test that could prove this. He decided to test for C-reactive protein (CRP), a molecule produced by the liver in response to an inflammatory signal. The higher the inflammation, the higher the level of CRP.[11]

Dr. Ridker succeeded in proving his theory and published it in the *New England Journal of Medicine* in 1997. He showed that people with high levels of CRP were three times as likely to die from a heart attack, regardless of their cholesterol levels. This revolutionized the concept of heart disease and all diseases. It is now accepted that atherosclerosis (hardening of the arteries) is actually an inflammatory disease.[12]

THE NEW MODEL OF HEART DISEASE

The new model of heart disease is based on both oxidation and inflammation. Although our body must have cholesterol to build healthy cells, high levels of LDL cholesterol can become oxidized by free radicals. The oxidized cholesterol triggers an inflammatory response that builds up white blood cells that turn into dangerous plaque, and damages the lining of the arteries. Damaged linings become sticky like Velcro and attract more oxidized cholesterol and white blood cells and cause more inflammation. It's a vicious cycle of oxidation, inflammation, white blood cells and plaque. Eventually the arteries become rigid and stiff and lined with plaque. A final inflammatory trigger causes plaque to tear off and a blood clot forms to repair the tear. That blood clot can occlude the circulation to the brain or the heart causing a stroke or a heart attack.

The latest research also shows that maintaining healthy levels of nitric oxide maintains a healthy arterial lining—the key to heart health. Nitric oxide also works in the mitochondria of all cells to maintain a healthy energy level.[13]

Lowering high levels of cholesterol is still important. Apparently, when an inflammatory reaction is occurring in the arteries, high levels of LDL cholesterol with certain "sticky" molecules attached cause higher levels of plaque to form and trigger even more inflammation in the artery wall. Controlling oxidation, inflammation and cholesterol and maintaining healthy levels of nitric oxide is the new model to prevent heart disease.

STATIN DRUGS LOWER CHOLESTEROL AND INFLAMMATION

Statin drugs that lower cholesterol are the most common prescription medication used to prevent heart attacks. Although doctors have mainly used statins to control cholesterol levels, they also lower inflammation—although they can have side effects. Studies using higher levels of statins show successful outcomes regarding coronary heart disease. Cholesterol lowering, however, will not make up for uncontrolled hypertension, smoking, high triglycerides, and obesity. These risks correlate with higher CRP levels, even if patients are treated with statins.

According to an editorial commentary on a statin study in the September, 2004, *Journal of the American Medical Association*, "This finding suggests an intriguing hypothesis, specifically, that the early benefits of statin therapy are derived largely from the anti-inflammatory effects of the drugs, whereas the delayed benefits are lipid-modulated." [14] Maintaining low levels of oxidation and inflammation and healthy levels of nitric oxide with natural substances is a healthier alternative for most people. Some people, however, will need to take statins, if tolerated.

For many years, the medical model of disease had been that each disease is a separate problem with a separate cause and specific medications for that disease. Due to Dr. Ridker's work with chronic inflammation and Dr. Harman's insight into oxidation, this is changing. The world of medical science is going through a radical upheaval in understanding the causes of most modern debilitating and "killer" diseases including heart disease, cancer, stroke, diabetes, Alzheimer's, arthritis, multiple sclerosis, fibromyalgia, chronic fatigue, allergies, and more. The two words that are rocking the previous model of medicine are inflammation and oxidation.

An article in *Time* magazine, February 23, 2004, said, "Instead of different treatments for, say, heart disease, Alzheimer's and colon cancer, there might be a single, inflammation-reducing remedy that would prevent all three." And, instead of relying on prescription medications and surgery to treat and manage the symptoms, we may be able to prevent these diseases with natural antioxidants, anti-inflammatories and supplements that maintain healthy levels of nitric oxide.

OXIDATION, BLOOD VESSELS AND AGING

Once again, the heart is in the center of it all. Doctors now know that it is the oxidation of cholesterol that is the problem. When cholesterol and other fats become oxidized, it starts a process of inflammation that leads to plaque and heart disease.

The role of free radicals in the health of blood vessels is particularly important. Blood vessels are absolutely critical to overall health because they supply oxygen and nutrients to cells throughout the body. Damage to blood vessels can have a profound impact on the heart and the brain and contribute to diseases associated with aging (e.g., diabetes, atherosclerosis, hypertension). The cells that line blood vessels, called endothelial cells, are vulnerable to damage from free radicals and inflammatory chemicals.

I want to emphasize the importance of the endothelial cells. This lining along our blood vessels is only one cell thick and therefore somewhat fragile. The supplements discussed in this book have very great health benefits for endothelial cells. They reduce inflammation and oxidation and increase nitric oxide. Aging blood vessels may be the primary factor in overall aging. If we can't get oxygen and nutrients to our cells, they begin to weaken and die. If there's not enough nitric oxide, they get rigid and stiff. If the endothelium gets stiff and rigid, we end up with high blood pressure. If the endothelium gets inflamed, it can trigger blood clots. Therapies that support the health of the endothelium and blood vessels could help maintain health throughout the body into old age.[15]

Researchers are now seeing the endothelial lining in all blood vessels as a key target for short- and long-term anti-inflammatory and antioxidant therapy. Initial studies showed that giving antioxidants improved blood flow in the brachial artery in patients with coronary heart disease or congestive heart failure.[16] Flavonoid and nonflavonoid polyphenols as found in red wine support the production of nitric oxide in the endothelial cells. Nitric oxide promotes relaxation of arteries and fights free radical damage to these delicate cells. Resveratrol, alpha lipoic acid, acetyl L-carnitine, quercetin, and red wine extract with 95% OPCs all protect the heart by reducing or preventing oxidation and inflammation and increasing nitric oxide.

ALL RISK FACTORS FOR CHRONIC DISEASES ARE ASSOCIATED WITH INFLAMMATION AND OXIDATION

Although I agree with almost all of the risk factors of the authorities, I think that the way they are presented is misleading. These are not separate risk factors. The root risk factors for all of them are chronic inflammation and oxidation.

Because scientists can more accurately identify markers of inflammation in the human body than they can oxidative stress, many of the studies below focus on identifying inflammation. Actually detecting levels of free radicals in the body is very difficult. However, electron spin resonance can detect the footprints of free radicals and scientists continue to develop new ways of identifying oxidative stress levels.[17][18]

Combined Risk Factors for Chronic Disease:
Smoking or environmental smoke. A study on aging, smoking and oxidative stress found that even if exposure to tobacco is stopped, inflammation persists, especially if the smoker is older. There is a growing body of evidence about damage from oxidative stress due to cigarette smoking. In smokers, one of the major antioxidants in the body, glutathione, becomes oxidized and accumulates in the lungs and overwhelms the body's antioxidant defenses. As smoke damages blood vessels, an immune response is triggered that increases inflammation.[19] Mitochondrial antioxidants like alpha lipoic acid can actually help repair smoke-damaged cells.[20]

Obesity. Obesity is a state of increased inflammation and oxidative stress. Obese humans also have increased oxidative stress in the endothelial lining.[21][22] By targeting oxidation and inflammation, we may be able to help reduce the incidence of type 2 diabetes associated with obesity. The recent research that showed resveratrol prevented diabetes in aging rats and studies that showed alpha lipoic acid reduced the symptoms of diabetic neuropathy in humans are very encouraging.[23]

Not exercising. High levels of exercise can initially increase oxidation. However, studies have shown that exercise also increases enzymes that produce antioxidants, leaving your body in better shape than before you exercised. Inactivity *increases* oxidative stress with no increased production of antioxidants, resulting in higher levels of oxidation.[24] I highly recommend regular, moderate exercise and antioxidants.

High stress. Researchers have established a link between stress, inflammation and disease. Individuals with major depression have a much higher inflammatory response to psychological stress than people who do not suffer from depression.[25] Antioxidant and anti-inflammatory supplements may help.

Diet low in fruits and vegetables. Studies have shown that people who ate a diet high in fruits, vegetables, nuts, olive oil and whole grains had significantly lower markers of inflammation than people who ate fewer fruits and vegetables. People who ate foods with higher levels of flavonoids, especially quercetin, a natural anti-inflammatory, had lower levels of chronic diseases, including lung cancer.[26 27 28] It is the high polyphenol antioxidants in fruits, vegetables, and red wine that are probably the main factors responsible for the healthy effects.[29]

Diet high in all types of fat. This has been disproven. It is the *kinds of fat* and other aspects of the diet that matter, not the total fat intake. A study published in 2007 compared the effects of a Mediterranean diet high in olive oil, walnuts, fruits and vegetables, with a low-fat diet. The randomized, controlled study included 9,000 high-risk participants with type 2 diabetes or three or more other risk factors for coronary heart disease. The main goal was to measure oxidation of LDL cholesterol as a risk for heart disease. Glucose levels, systolic blood pressure and total cholesterol/HDL cholesterol ratios, and inflammation were also measured. The results showed high levels of virgin olive oil *reduced* oxidized LDL. The two Mediterranean diet groups had lower glucose levels, lower systolic blood pressure, lower inflammation, and better HDL ratios. The Mediterranean diet with olive oil reduced oxidized LDL by 10.6; with walnuts reduced it 7.3; a low fat diet only reduced it by 2.9. This showed a clear anti-oxidant benefit from a diet high in olive oil, walnuts, fruits and vegetables. It also showed that a low-fat diet does not, by itself, lower a primary marker of heart disease.[30]

Diet high in saturated fat and cholesterol. Saturated fats and cholesterol are the most controversial risk factors. Not all saturated fat is the same and they have very different biochemical effects on our tissues. The type of saturated fat in chocolate (stearic acid), for example, is a healthy fat. Some types of saturated fat, however, when combined with high LDL cholesterol increase inflammation. Good saturated fats and bad saturated fats can exist within the same foods. However, adding olive oil, avocadoes, red wine, and fruits high in antioxidants to the meal helps counter the negative effects of bad saturated fats. Olive oil, especially, interferes with the inflammation response. It's the combination of foods that we eat that makes the biggest difference.

As I mentioned in an earlier chapter, the long-term dietary studies do not support a connection between high dietary saturated fat and cholesterol with higher levels of heart disease. Some studies have shown that saturated fat raised inflammation levels a modest amount; others found that it did not raise inflammation. One study found that eating four eggs a day increased inflammation in lean, healthy subjects but not in obese insulin resistant subjects. A study at Harvard found no correlation between eating eggs and levels of cholesterol.[31] Research did show that eating lean red meat did not raise inflammation levels.[32] Without going into all of the details of all of the studies, I conclude that common sense and the latest research are your best guides.

Based on research and common sense, I believe we can enjoy meals with moderate amounts of lean red meat (preferably pasture raised instead of corn fed because corn increases proinflammatory molecules in meat) and whole dairy products and eggs from healthy sources. Eating fruits, vegetables, olive oil and nuts creates a healthy, balanced diet. Having a glass of wine or another beverage, food, or herb with high levels of antioxidants helps lower the natural rise in oxidative stress after a meal.[33] This is the traditional French way of eating.

Diet high in trans fats. Many studies have shown trans fats to be inflammatory. Trans fats also raise serum levels of LDL (bad) cholesterol, reduce levels of HDL (good) cholestrol, and increase the oxidation of cholesterol.[34] The Food and Drug Administraton has stated that there is no safe level of trans fats in a healthy diet.

Diet high in sugar and refined carbohydrates. According to a study by Simin Liu, M.D., Ph.D. at Harvard Medical School, women eating diets that included potatoes, breakfast cereals, white bread, muffins and white rice had elevated CRP levels of inflammation.[35] High consumption of refined sugar may also promote inflammation, according to new research published in the *American Journal of Clinical Nutrition.*[36]

High levels of salt. High levels of salt activate inflammatory cytokines and drive oxidative stress that contributes to salt-sensitive high blood pressure.[37 38] Processed foods and food eaten in restaurants contribute most of the salt you eat. You may think you are not consuming a high level of salt because you never add salt to your food. However, if you eat out frequently or eat canned and processed foods, you may be getting much more salt than you think.

Diabetes. Obesity is often associated with diabetes and a state of chronic low-level inflammation. Increased glucose metabolism can lead to a rise in mitochondrial production of free radicals creating oxidative stress. A recent study says, "The evidence strongly suggests that type 2 diabetes is an inflammatory disease and that inflammation is a primary cause of obesity-linked insulin resistance, hyperglycemia and high cholesterol rather than merely a consequence." [39]

High cholesterol or abnormal blood lipids. The oxidation of lipids in high levels of LDL cholesterol triggers inflammation leading to lesions. Enzymes associate with HDL may protect against oxidation. [40]

High blood pressure. High blood pressure is also strongly associated with inflammation and oxidative stress. [41] Nitric oxide generated by antioxidants found in

---

Common Causes of Inflammation and Oxidation

- Body's own mitochondrial energy production
- Obesity
- Stress
- Vitamin and mineral deficiencies
- Bacteria, viruses, candida, parasites
- Trans fats
- Indoor and outdoor pollution
- High levels of refined flour and sugar
- Smoking
- Sleep deprivation
- Household cleaning supplies, weed/ bug killers
- Chemicals in cosmetics

The 5 Worst Inflammatory Foods

1. French fries
2. Donuts
3. Sodas
4. Chips
5. Chicken nuggets fried in trans fats

red wine and other sources, is critical to maintaining normal blood pressure. Nitric oxide helps relax arteries, lowers blood pressure, and prevents and restores damage to the endothelial lining.[42]

It's clear that inflammation and oxidation are at the core of chronic diseases and aging. However, in order to truly understand how we can stay healthy as we age, we need to understand where oxidation starts—inside our mitochondria.

4
MITOCHONDRIA—MIGHTY DISEASE FIGHTERS HOLD THE KEY TO THE FOUNTAIN OF YOUTH

Once again, the story of a major breakthrough in modern science begins with one person and a moment of brilliant insight. Dr. Denham Harman had worked for nearly 15 years for the Shell Oil Company studying free radical chemistry in relation to the oil industry. One day in the 1950s, his wife gave him an article to read about aging. Something in the article inspired him and he says that this was the beginning of his quest to find the one common cause of aging.

Dr. Harman left the oil industry and attended medical school at Stanford and then joined the Donner Laboratory of Medical Physics at the University of California, Berkeley. At that point, says Dr. Harman in a speech at the 2nd Annual Monaco Anti-Aging Conference, "I settled down to the problem of what causes aging and what can we do about it." [1] [2]

THE FREE RADICAL THEORY OF AGING

According to Dr. Harman's account, he became frustrated. He says that he could not find the one thing that would account for aging. He was at the point of giving up when a phrase just floated across his mind—*free radicals*. He knew he had found what he had been looking for.

Dr. Harman, of course, wanted to share this tremendous insight with his colleagues, so he says he walked around the campus at U.C. Berkeley and talked to people about his idea that free radicals could be the primary cause of aging. Only two people thought there might be something in it. Dr. Harman knew he was going to have to present a published paper to get anyone to believe in his theory. In 1956, he published, "Aging: a theory based on free radical and radiation chemistry," in the *Journal of Gerontology*, and it received a great deal of publicity. It became known as The Free Radical Theory of Aging.

Before Dr. Harman published his new theory, anti-aging was hardly recognized as science. It was in the realm of the "kooks" and science fiction. By proposing a valid, scientific cause for the aging process, Dr. Harman opened the door to other scientists to solve one of the great mysteries of humankind—what can we do to stay healthy as we age and even extend the number of years we live.

This research has continued up to the present when scientists have discovered several crucial antioxidant compounds like resveratrol, alpha lipoic acid, red wine extract, and quercetin that may help us maintain good health into old age.

THE   KEY TO AGING AND DISEASE—THE MITOCHONDRIA

In 1972, Dr. Harman published a new paper, "A biologic clock: the mitochondria?" in the *Journal of the American Geriatric Society* that revised his previous theory. Dr. Harman now believed that protecting our *mitochondria* from free radical damage was the key to preventing aging. According to Dr. Harman, the scientific community was not that interested in his new theory about mitochondria called The Mitochondrial Theory of Aging. He had to wait for growth in the mitochrondria field.

In 1980, Dr. J. Miquel published a follow-up paper supporting the importance of the mitochondria in the aging process. It still didn't catch on. It wasn't until 1989, when Dr. A.W. Linnane and his colleagues in Melbourne, Australia, published another paper on mitochondria and aging that the scientific community started to recognize that the mitochondria could be the key to staying healthy as we age.

WHAT ARE MITOCHONDRIA?

Deep inside almost every cell in your body are tiny structures called mitochondria (mite-oh-con-dree-ah). There may be thousands of these tiny structures (also called organelles) inside one cell. Organs that require the most energy, such as the heart and brain, have the most mitochondria—up to 7,000 mitochondria in one heart cell! Scientists theorize that mitochondria evolved first and then cells engulfed them.

Mitochondria were discovered in the 1950s with the electron microscope that could see into the inside of the cell. Scientists were amazed to find out that mitochondria contained their own DNA. The cells have nuclear DNA and mitochondria have DNA as well. Once mitochondria were discovered, researchers had to find out what role they played in the body. The answer was astounding— mitochondria produce 95% of the body's total energy! One of the first scientists to study mitochondria called them the body's "power plants." [3]

In the process of creating all this energy from oxygen, mitochondria also produce free radicals that can damage the DNA of the mitochondria. As we age, this damage accumulates, reducing the ability of the mitochondria to function and keep on creating energy. Plus, poorly functioning mitochondria create higher and higher levels of free radicals that cause oxidative damage to the cells in the body leading to disease and aging. Research has shown that mitochondrial DNA damage increases with age.[4]

HOW DO THEY WORK?

Researchers soon discovered that mitochondria transform the oxygen we breathe into energy, a process using adenosine triphosphate or ATP. No mitochondria, no energy. Healthy mitochondria, lots of energy. During the time that mitochondria and ATP were discovered, Dr. Denham Harman published his paper which became known as The Free Radical Theory of Aging. He theorized that it was the oxidation of molecules in the body that caused damage to cells, deterioration, chronic diseases and aging. In 1972 He amended this theory to The Mitochondrial Theory of Aging. He believed that it was the oxidation *inside the mitochondria* that results in damage to the DNA and the ultimate deterioration and destruction of cells in the heart, brain, liver, skeletal muscle and other organs that lead to chronic disease and eventually death. If we could keep our mitochondria and its DNA healthy— how long could we live and how healthy would we be?

WHAT CAUSES OXIDATION INSIDE MITOCHONDRIA?

In the process of producing energy, free radicals are

produced within the mitochondria. Fortunately, most of these free radicals are kept under control by the mitochondrial "police force"—mitochondrial antioxidants. There's one real nasty free radical molecule inside mitochondria called superoxide anion. You need a lot of antioxidant power to make sure that one doesn't cause problems. However, if your mitochondrial antioxidants are low or weak, superoxide anion and other free radicals get the upper hand and get out of control leading to DNA damage and ultimately damage to cells, tissues and organs. It was first believed there were only oxygen free radicals. Now we know there are also nitrogen free radicals. In fact, when a nitrogen free radical combines with superoxide anion it makes one of the most toxic free radicals known— the really bad guy, peroxynitrate. The technical term used by scientists for all free radicals is RONS—reactive oxygen and nitrogen species, but most people still call them free radicals.

IT'S THE DNA

Scientists now agree with Dr. Harman's theory that it is the vulnerable DNA within the mitochondria that must be protected from damage. The nuclear DNA is much more stable, probably because the process of producing energy is not happening right next to the nuclear DNA. It's like having a fire next door to you—if that fire gets out of control, it could damage your yard or your house. If that fire is down the street, you're in a lot less danger.[5] As we get older, the DNA damage begins to accumulate and the mitochondria doesn't function as well. It makes sense that if the vitality center of the body—the mitochondria—is damaged, you will have less energy, less ability to withstand stress, and less ability to recover if you become sick. All of this brings about the deteriorating state of health and the lower levels of energy and functioning we call "aging" and chronic disease.

For some time it was believed that the mitochondrial DNA did not have a natural repair system. Fortunately, we now know that mitochondria are capable of repairing oxidative damage to their DNA! This is important because if the DNA is damaged then it spreads the damage. The defective cell is duplicated over and over as the cells divide, thus allowing the damaged cells to multiply. This replication of damaged cells may lead to cancer. Damaged mitochondria also produce more free radicals leading to a vicious cycle of destruction.

MITOCHONDRIA AND ANTI-AGING

Not only did Dr. Linnane and others observe the deterioration of mitochondria in the laboratory due to free radicals, Dr. Linnane also demonstrated that only 5% of a ninety-year-old's mitochondrial DNA from skeletal muscle tissue was still undamaged. Ninety-five percent was damaged! One of the most observable effects of aging—and one of the hardest to prevent—is muscle deterioration. You can exercise and work out with weights, which is helpful in maintaining good muscle tone, but you have to start in the mitochondria to really make a difference.

Mitochondrial DNA in heart, brain, and skeletal muscle appears to deteriorate the most—the deterioration increasing exponentially after the age of 30 or 40.[6] All of the mitochondria of a five-year-old produce equal amounts of energy. However, after about the age of 40, we begin to see a huge change in mitochondria with some cells still producing energy and others losing steam, while others aren't functioning at all. This can vary widely among individuals, which is why some people are obviously aging more quickly than others—they have more oxidation damage to their mitochondria. In a paper published in 1995, Linnane called this "the theory of universality of bioenergetic disease."[7]

MITOCHONDRIA—THE SECRET OF LIFE *AND* DEATH

Mitochondria and its effect on aging was very exciting news for scientists and for the general public. It appeared that the actual mystery of aging was being revealed for the first time. Once scientists understood what caused aging, then perhaps something could be done about it. Then more big news was announced. Not only were mitochondria the energy power house of the body—the source of life—they were responsible for the organized *death* of cells as well. It is part of the normal functioning of the body that cells have a normal life span. They live and they die. You want damaged or weak cells with damaged DNA to die so that they do not continue to replicate more weak and damaged cells, a process that leads to cancer. Nature designed a way for weak and damaged cells to be disposed of properly. That process is called apoptosis (ay-pop-toe-sis), also called "cell suicide," and it is controlled by the mitochondria.

Mitochondria regulate an orderly death for weak or diseased cells by opening up a "megachannel" in its membrane that triggers the cell to self destruct. If enough mitochondria perceive there is a problem and open up this channel, the cell dies. This contains the process within the cell and doesn't damage nearby cells. It's nice and tidy.

Healthy mitochondria create healthy vitality and they also create an orderly process of cell death—both are necessary for the total health of the body.

MITOCHONDRIA AND CHRONIC DISEASES

Cancer—Mitochondria in the News!

Mitochondria are the *big* news in cancer research, even though most cancer researchers have not been focusing on this part of the cell. At the 2005 meeting of the American Association for Cancer Research, leading cancer researcher Gerard Evan, Ph.D., admitted, "I had to be brought kicking and screaming into mitochondria." He said that he and other cancer researchers who had ignored the processes of the mitochondria can't ignore it any longer. Other cancer researchers are starting to take notice because, said Evan, "All roads lead to the mitochondria."[8]

The reason for this interest in mitochondria by cancer researchers is new discoveries about how tumors grow. Tumors take a lot of energy to grow and instead of using the mitochondrial process that uses ATP to produce energy, they use a "back-up" system called glycolosis that uses only sugar, instead of oxygen and sugar, to produce energy. It was thought the reason tumor cells did this was because the mitochondrial system was too damaged by the cancer to produce energy. It was also thought that because the mitochondria was damaged it no longer had the ability to regulate apoptosis and kill off cancer cells. However, research published in 2006 by Craig Thompson, M.D., at the University of Pennsylvania revealed that if the back-up sugar system is suppressed, the mitochondrial system of producing energy will kick back in.[9]

Then, in early 2007, researchers at the University of

Alberta in Canada, led by Dr. Evangelos Michelakis, discovered that a simple molecule called dichloroacetate (DCA) that has been used for decades to treat genetic mitochondrial disease, reduced tumor size in animals up to 70% by restarting mitochondrial ATP production. Dr. Michelakis' research showed that DCA switched the energy that fueled cancer cells from glycolosis back to the mitochondria. *The normalization of mitochondrial function resulted in a significant decrease in tumor growth* in test tube and animal models. The cancer tumors just withered. Plus, unlike most cancer drugs, DCA did not have any effects on normal, noncancerous tissues. Dr. Michelakis believes that by restarting the mitochondrial energy process, the mitochondria also restarts the process of apoptosis that kills off the cancer cells, restricting the ability of tumors to continue growing.

Dr. Michelakis also noted that DCA may be effective against a wide variety of cancers because the suppression of normal mitochondrial function is common to all forms of cancer.[10]

It's possible that oxidative damage may trigger the initial dysfunction in the mitochondria that shuts down the normal apoptosis function. This may then initiate the switch to the alternate energy supply of glycolysis that fuels the cancer growth without the check of apoptosis from normal mitochondrial functioning.[11][12]

The research in this field is very exciting and I expect to see more in-depth research into cancer and mitochondria in the near future and clinical benefits within a few years. Meanwhile, by supplying the body with plenty of mitochondrial antioxidants like alpha lipoic acid and resveratrol, we may be able to keep the mitochondrial system functioning at a healthy level and avoid the unchecked development of cancerous cells.

Heart Disease and Mitochondria

Heart cells are composed of 70% mitochondria. If something is going wrong with the mitochondria in your heart, you are going to feel it. Clay F. Semenkovich, M.D. at the Washington University School of Medicine and his colleagues reported in research published in the May, 2005, edition of *Nature* that failures in the mitochondria due to aging are the prime suspects for atherosclerosis and heart disease.

Atherosclerosis and Mitochondria

Hardening and clogging of the arteries may occur in nonsmokers who have *low* levels of LDL cholesterol. Smoking and high LDL cholesterol have been considered two of the primary risk factors for atherosclerosis. Therefore, there must be other factors involved. Recent research has identified chronic inflammation and oxidation as the two consistent factors for heart disease.

Now, Dr. Semenkovich and his colleagues have evidence that in heart disease as in cancer "all roads lead to the mitochondria." His team discovered that a failure of mitochondrial production of energy in the aging artery walls creates inflammation that leads to hardening and clogging of arteries. One solution, according to researchers in this field, would be to supply the mitochondria with antioxidants to reduce free radicals and inflammation. Healthy mitochondria would reduce damage by free radicals to the arteries.[13]

Other researchers agree. Age-related oxidative stress in the mitochondria may be at the root of heart failure according to a study published in late 2006 in the *Journal of Biological Chemistry*. This study showed conclusively that oxidative stress caused specific changes in the mitochondria leading to excessive oxidation, lowered production of ATP energy, and reduced ability of the heart to contract normally. Administration of an antioxidant normally produced in the mitochondria (superoxide dismutase) significantly reduced the symptoms. The results of this study showed that oxygen free radicals produced in the mitochondria play a pivotal role in the development and progression of heart failure, and that antioxidants can make a difference.[14]

Heart Attacks and Mitochondria

Dr. Mark Sussman, head of the Heart Institute at San Diego State University, was awarded a $9.5 million grant in 2006 to study how protecting the mitochondria can preserve cells during a heart attack. "Mitochondria, a cell's energy center, are the key to a heart's survival during a heart attack," he said in a press release. Scientists want to prevent the damage from a heart attack by supporting the mitochondria before and after a heart attack occurs.[15] The use of resveratrol, and other antioxidants that can penetrate into the mitochondria, shows great promise for pre- and post-conditioning to reduce the damage by heart attacks.[16 17] I will cover this more in Chapter 6.

An important study on acute heart attacks revealed that heart attack patients have about half the normal levels of antioxidants such as glutathione, vitamin C and E, "indicating severe damage to the antioxidant system, which is unable to combat oxidative stress and inflammation."[18] Supplementing with mitochondrial antioxidants may be vital to restoring health after a heart attack.

Diabetes and Mitochondria

Researchers have also discovered that mitochondrial dysfunction plays a major role in insulin resistance and possibly the development of type 2 diabetes. One study compared young and elderly participants who were of similar body types. They all had similar levels of fat and lean body muscle. Everyone in the study was nonsmoking, didn't exercise much, and had no history of diabetes or high blood pressure. The first test showed that the older people were already relatively insulin resistant compared to the younger people in the study—even though there were no clinical signs of diabetes.

Plus, the researchers found that the insulin resistance was located mainly in the muscle tissue attached to bones, called skeletal muscle. The researchers evaluated the rates of mitochondrial energy production in the skeletal muscle tissue and discovered that the *healthy production of energy by mitochondria was 40% less in the elderly*. There was obviously an age-related reduction of mitochondrial function and/ or number that contributed to insulin resistance that could possibly lead to type 2 diabetes. Earlier I noted that skeletal muscle tissue has an especially high level of mitochondrial problems as people age.[19]

That higher levels of mitochondrial antioxidants make a difference in healthy organ function is shown in the liver. There is less damage to mitochondria in the liver than in other organs of the body, even in the livers of rats with diabetes. The researchers said that this was due to the higher levels of the antioxidants that accumulate in the liver. Liver antioxidants like glutathione help protect against mitochondria damage.[20]

The Brain and Mitochondria

Losing one's memory, foggy thinking, and lack of skill in doing things are some of the most common symptoms of aging. One survey found that seniors dreaded losing their memory more than dying. The research is showing that brain mitochondria is closely connected to aging and brain function. In animal studies, researchers found that antioxidant activity in the brain mitochondria decreased up to 78% as animals aged. As the oxidation increased, enzyme activity that creates antioxidants decreased. The higher the level of antioxidant enzymes, the better the mice in the study performed on memory and coordination tests. The researchers concluded that the declining energy supply in the brain mitochondria was a factor in problems of memory and coordination that are often associated with aging.[21] Acetyl L-carnitine and alpha lipoic acid play a critical role in providing the mitochondria with the fuel it needs to create energy in the brain.

Brain tissue in the hippocampus, the part of the brain most susceptible to stress, has a slow turnover of mitochondria. This slow turnover allows it to accumulate more DNA-damaged mitochondria as people age, leading to more neurological damage.[22] High levels of antioxidants in the brain may help clean out damaged mitochondria.

MITOCHONDRIAL ANTIOXIDANTS ARE MORE THAN FREE RADICAL FIGHTERS

We mainly think of antioxidants as the molecules that fight the oxidizing free radicals. But scientists are discovering that antioxidants have many more jobs that they do in the body. We are learning more every day. For some years it was believed that acetyl L-carnitine was a mitochondrial antioxidant. Now, the research by Drs. Bruce Ames and Tory Hagen at Berkeley has shown that it is an important supplier of fuel to the mitochondria, but it is not an antioxidant.[23] Alpha lipoic acid, however, is the key mitochondrial antioxidant.

At this time, we know that mitochondrial antioxidants like alpha lipoic acid, resveratrol and quercetin, plus fuel supplier acetyl L-carnitine

- Quench free radicals that damage mitochondrial DNA
- Reduce inflammation
- Trigger genes to do the right thing and not the wrong thing
- Stimulate regeneration of nerves
- Transport vital amino acids into the cells
- Bring fuel into the mitochondria
- Take out the garbage from the mitochondria
- Prevent damage to the mitochondria by free radicals that follows a lack of oxygen from heart attacks and strokes
- Increase the number of mitochondria and the energy production of the mitochondria
- Support the mitochondrial production of nitric oxide that keeps blood vessels healthy
- Help all the important antioxidants stay in the game by recycling each other

MITOCHONDRIAL ANTIOXIDANTS TO THE RESCUE

Some of you may remember the bumper stickers that were common a few years back. Save the Whales. Save the Seals. Save the Redwoods. I'm going to propose a new bumper sticker—Save the Mitochondria! Mitochondria are more important than any other living organism to our health and well being. The more I research, the more I am convinced that maintaining strong and healthy mitochondria is the key to living a long and healthy life without chronic illness. The big question is, how do we do it?

Fortunately, there are sound scientific strategies of using specific antioxidants, minerals, vitamins, and anti-inflammatory supplements that decrease age-related mitochondrial damage from oxidative stress. Alpha lipoic acid, acetyl L-carnitine, resveratrol, red wine extract with 95% OPCs, quercetin and other supplements can support healthy mitochondria—they are the secret to living a long and healthy life.

5
ALPHA LIPOIC ACID AND ACETYL L-CARNITINE— A SUPER ANTIOXIDANT TEAMS UP WITH AN ENERGY POWERHOUSE TO REVERSE AGING

That maintaining healthy mitochondria results in healthy aging is becoming more and more apparent. The most useful antioxidants are those that act directly to protect the mitochondria and keep it supplied with fuel. Alpha lipoic acid and acetyl L-carnitine work together to make sure that mitochondria are protected and have plenty of fuel to make energy. They are two of mitochondria's best friends.

The antioxidants that protect the mitochondria are not lone rangers. It is now accepted that antioxidants work best when they work together. There is an "antioxidant buddy system" that brings several antioxidants together to work as a team to support the mitochondria. Members of the team help each other stay in the game of fighting free radicals. If one antioxidant has an electron snatched by a free radical, then another member of the team will replace it. This is called recycling. Alpha lipoic acid is the only known player that can recycle *all* of the other mitochondrial antioxidants.[1]

WHAT IS ALPHA LIPOIC ACID?

This compound was a mystery when it was first discovered in the late 1930s. It didn't even have a name. Scientists just knew that "something" enhanced the growth of bacterial cells. In 1951, biochemist Lester Reed isolated 30 milligrams of lipoic acid from 10 tons of beef. Scientists now had a name for it, but they really didn't know what it did. It wasn't until 1989 that alpha lipoic acid was discovered to be a powerful antioxidant. Two years later, the research team of Dr. Lester Packer at the University of California, Berkeley, discovered that it might be the most powerful antioxidant of all! It's so powerful that it is now called the "Universal Antioxidant." Not only did Dr. Packer discover the power of alpha lipoic acid, he and his team were the first to acknowledge that antioxidants communicated with each other and worked as a team—with alpha lipoic acid being the most important member of the mitochondrial team.[2]

WHAT'S SPECIAL ABOUT ALPHA LIPOIC ACID?

Unlike every other antioxidant, alpha lipoic acid can work as a free radical scavenger in the outside membrane of mitochondria that is made of fat, and penetrate into the watery interior environment of the mitochondria. It is both fat and water soluble. No other antioxidant is both. It can also cross the blood-brain barrier. So that makes it a very valuable player. It can track down free radicals wherever they go. Alpha lipoic acid helps its team members vitamins C, E, coenzyme Q-10, and glutathione conserve antioxidant resources. Alpha lipoic acid helps regenerate all of the most important mitochondrial antioxidants after they've been slugging it out with free radicals and have been weakened by the fight. It's the best antioxidant buddy there is.

When the important mitochondrial antioxidants (co-enzyme Q-10, glutathione, vitamins C and E) find a free radical and deactivate it by giving it an electron, these antioxidants become weak free radicals themselves. They've lost an electron and cannot go after any more free radicals. They're kind of like the wounded players on a team, having to sit on the sidelines. Alpha lipoic acid can change that. Alpha lipoic acid can donate electrons to all of these key players and bring them back into the game. It regenerates them. It can even regenerate itself. It's the only antioxidant that can do that.[3]

Other antioxidants can act as buddies as well. Vitamin C can recycle E and E can recycle C. These are all "buddy antioxidants." But alpha lipoic acid is the only known antioxidant that can regenerate the most important mitochondrial antioxidant of all—glutathione.

GLUTATHIONE'S BEST BUDDY

Glutathione is made in the heart of the mitochondria. It is the primary antioxidant that keeps free radicals from damaging our power center because it is made inside every cell in the body. Maintaining a high level of glutathione in our cells is vital to the body's survival. Glutathione is the master detoxifier. It keeps the liver detoxifying all the pollutants and poisons we are normally exposed to. If your liver is overwhelmed with a poison and uses up all of your glutathione trying to detoxify the poison, you will die.

The problem is, we cannot supplement glutathione directly. The molecule is too big to permeate the cell membrane and into the mitochondria. There are two ways to keep glutathione active in the antioxidant game. One is to provide the ingredients, called precursors, that make up glutathione. The other way is to have enough alpha lipoic acid to keep recycling glutathione. In further support of the benefit of alpha lipoic acid in reducing free radicals, a recent study showed that alpha lipoic acid helped maintain normal levels of glutathione after periods of intense exercise that cause free radicals to rise.[4]

ALPHA LIPOIC ACID SAVES THE LIVER FROM POISON

The importance of alpha lipoic acid to the detoxification process of glutathione in the liver was dramatically revealed in the 1970s. A young doctor who had previously studied mushrooms was in the emergency room when a couple was brought in who had eaten the deadly amanita mushroom. They were given no chance to live. The young physician, Dr. Burt Berkson, remembered reading about an experimental compound being used in Germany for mushroom poisoning. He called the National Institutes of Health (NIH) and they had some of this compound on hand. It was alpha lipoic acid. They overnighted some to Dr. Berkson who gave it intravenously to the couple. They both lived. The alpha lipoic acid restored enough glutathione to detoxify and regenerate the livers of the patients.

It was mushroom season and the next week another couple was admitted with the same mushroom poisoning. The hospital authorities told Dr. Berkson not to use alpha lipoic acid again because it was an unproven substance. Dr. Berkson refused to follow those orders and gave alpha lipoic acid to the couple. Soon after he administered the alpha lipoic acid, the patients began to get better. They went home after ten days. Dr Berkson says he would have been fired, but the NIH took an interest and supported him. He has continued to champion alpha lipoic acid for acute liver poisoning, as a treatment for hepatitis C, and as a supplement to support our vital mitochondria.[5]

Dr. Packer was the first to actually prove in the laboratory that giving alpha lipoic acid raised levels of glutathione. In his first experiment, he added alpha lipoic acid to human and animal cells in tissue culture and the cellular levels of glutathione increased an amazing 30%! He had established that alpha lipoic acid recycled glutathione. Dr. Packer then did an experiment with animals. He added alpha lipoic acid to the food of rats. Levels of glutathione increased in the lungs, liver and blood of these animals. This was important because it showed that glutathione rose in the cells of organs where it could help prevent free radical damage.[6]

A Phase I Clinical Trial with patients who had chronic hepatitis C showed that those who received a combination of antioxidants that included alpha lipoic acid had significant improvement. Normalization of liver enzymes occurred in 44% of patients who had elevated pretreatment levels. These levels remained normal throughout the follow-up period in nearly 73%.[7] Alpha lipoic acid is so important that we manufacture it in every cell in our body. However, as we age, we manufacture less and less of it. And that's why I believe a supplement of alpha lipoic acid belongs in every anti-aging program.

ALPHA LIPOIC ACID HELPS MITOCHONDRIA MAKE ENERGY—ESPECIALLY AS WE AGE

In order to produce energy, mitochondria have to have the right kind of fuel. Alpha lipoic acid breaks down

sugar in a special way so that it can be used by the mitochondria to make energy. Without alpha lipoic acid, mitochondria will not get enough fuel and won't be able to
make energy. Eventually the cells will shut down. You've
learned that as we age, the mitochondria become less efficient in producing energy. We feel less vital and get tired
more easily. Without enough energy, the cells in our heart,
brain, liver and muscles get weaker and weaker until they
become diseased. As long as you have enough alpha lipoic acid, it will help the mitochondria maintain a high
level of energy. Alpha lipoic acid helps make the fuel that
runs the mitochondrial power plants of the body—and it
protects the mitochondria from free radical damage.

Alpha lipoic acid and acetyl L-carnitine have been
the focus of another brilliant scientist at U.C. Berkeley,
Dr. Bruce Ames. Dr. Ames became famous for devising a
simple test that identified substances that caused cancer.
He also showed that chemicals cause cancer by damaging
genes—something we take for granted now, but it was big
news back in the 1950s. His work on cancer caused him
to start looking at the role of free radicals. Free radicals
break strands of DNA and some of these breaks can cause
mutations that lead to cancer. He also noted that most
cancers increase with age. Ames thought that perhaps the
age-related increase in cancer might have something to
do with the rise in free radicals and oxidative stress damage that also increases with age. First he had to prove that
oxidation does increase with age.

Dr. Ames and his colleagues at Berkeley managed to
do that in 1990. They published evidence that they found
twice as much oxidation of DNA in two-year-old rats as
those in two-month-old rats. This encouraged Dr. Ames
to find out where the increase in free radicals was coming
from, and that took him to the mitochondria. "All roads

lead to the mitochondria" was turning out to be true again.

Dr. Ames thought that if he could intervene in the mitochondria and somehow reduce the oxidation level, he might be able to actually intervene in the aging process. He and his colleague, Dr. Tory Hagen, studied the changes that occur in the mitochondria of aging rats. Their landmark research discovered that old mitochondria are less efficient, they create less energy, and they make a lot more oxidants and free radicals. He found that Italian researchers were feeding acetyl L-carnitine to old rats to improve the function of their mitochondria. That made sense because carnitine helps transport fuel to the mitochondria. Ames started feeding acetyl L-carnitine to his old rats. Within weeks, he and Hagen noticed that the rats were more active. However, they were still producing a lot of oxidants—even a little more than before.[8]

Ames pondered on what he could do about the oxidation and came up with alpha lipoic acid—known as the best mitochondrial antioxidant. He added both acetyl L-carnitine and alpha lipoic acid to the diet of the old rats and the results were dramatic. In Ames' words, "Those old rats stood up and did the Macarena!"[9] Free radicals and oxidation damage to the mitochondria dropped dramatically. Skeletal muscle improved and the rat's activity levels doubled.[10] Hagen and another researcher, Dr. Jiankang Liu, tested the brain function of old rats. After just one month of taking acetyl L-carnitine and alpha lipoic acid, old rats' memory and coordination improved. Once again, the key was to provide the mitochondria with the fuel and antioxidants it needed to function at an efficient capacity.[11]

Ames is also a supporter of taking multivitamin and mineral supplements to insure that all the trace minerals and vitamins are available to support the mitochondria.

He emphasizes that the amount of micronutrients that is truly "required" is the amount needed to minimize DNA damage and oxidation damage in the mitochondria, not the amount needed to prevent acute deficiency disease. Ames cites several studies that show Americans are deficient in critical vitamins and minerals. He also emphasizes that the requirements for older people will be different than those of younger people.[12]

ALPHA LIPOIC ACID HELPS GENES DO THE RIGHT THING

Alpha lipoic acid also helps block the activation of bad genes. Certain genes have to be activated to work properly. For example, the genes that make us grow are activated when we are young, but then are deactivated at a certain age. However, free radicals can activate genes in a way that causes trouble. All antioxidants can help our DNA stay healthy by protecting it from free radical damage. However, alpha lipoic acid has a special role to play in controlling certain factors that cause genes to go bad.[13]

ALPHA LIPOIC ACID HAS STUNNING SUCCESS IN TREATING DIABETIC NEUROPATHY

Alpha lipoic acid has been used to alleviate one of the most disastrous side effects of diabetes—damage to the blood vessels and nerves, especially in the hands and feet, and the excruciating pain and debilitation it causes. Too often, diabetes is just seen as a "sugar problem." Diabetes damages the arteries and blood vessels, big and small, that circulate a healthy blood supply throughout the body. Without blood, the nerves die a painful death.

Without a good blood supply, serious infections can occur, especially in the feet. Eventually, these complications can lead to amputations. As the small blood vessels are damaged, it can lead to damage to the eyes and blindness. As the large blood vessels are damaged, it results in heart disease, heart attacks, and strokes. Damage to the nerves caused by diabetes is called diabetic neuropathy.

A ground-breaking double-blind, placebo-controlled study in 1997 of over 300 patients on the effect of alpha lipoic acid (also called thioctic acid by scientists) on diabetic peripheral nerve damage and heart damage found that intravenous alpha lipoic acid significantly reduced the symptoms of pain, burning, nerve irritation, and numbness. Two out of four indications of heart problems were improved. The researchers concluded that intravenous treatment with alpha lipoic acid (600 mg/day) over three weeks is safe and effective in reducing symptoms of diabetic peripheral neuropathy, and oral treatment with 800 mg/day for four months may improve cardiac autonomic dysfunction. There were no significant adverse affects.[14]

In 2004, a review was done of all the best studies using alpha lipoic acid to treat diabetic neuropathy. This review concluded that oxidative stress from free radicals may be the fundamental cause of diabetic neuropathy and that alpha lipoic acid addressed this problem. This analysis included the largest sample of diabetic patients (1258) ever studied with any type of drug to reduce symptoms of diabetic neuropathy. It concluded that intravenous alpha lipoic acid for three weeks at the dosages above reduced the horrible pain and disability of neuropathy and also helped to solve the underlying problem—not just treat the symptoms. It also concluded that oral alpha lipoic acid for three to four months also helped restore healthy heart function. If you have diabetic neuropathy, show this to your doctor. Alpha lipoic acid is a safe and effective treatment.[15]

A more recent study found that once-daily *oral* doses of 600 mg of alpha lipoic acid for five weeks also worked to reduce symptoms of diabetic neuropathy. There was significant improvement for stabbing and burning pain. Higher dosages than 600 mg sometimes resulted in nausea, vomiting and vertigo.[16]

It has been noted that diabetes patients have low levels of glutathione. Without enough glutathione, there's not enough energy to heal the cells and keep free radicals from continually damaging tissue. Once again, we see that the key to preventing major damage from diabetes lies in the tiny power centers of the body—the mitochondria. Alpha lipoic acid is one of the main players that keeps levels of glutathione high and the mitochondria going strong.[17]

ALPHA LIPOIC ACID COMPLETELY PREVENTS INCREASE IN ATHEROSCLEROSIS

Another terrible consequence of diabetes is that it dramatically increases your chance of having heart disease. It makes sense. High levels of insulin damage the endothelial lining, increasing inflammation, the build up of plaque, and heart disease. High insulin levels damage arteries, capillaries and nerves. Alpha lipoic acid can help. Once you understand that the underlying cause of all of these chronic diseases is inflammation and oxidation, especially in the mitochondria, then it makes sense that if you have one chronic disease, you have a greater chance of having other chronic diseases. And if you find a way to prevent oxidation and inflammation, it will help all the cells in your body. That's why alpha lipoic acid is called the "Universal Antioxidant"—it helps the mitochondria throughout your entire body.

A recent study reports that giving alpha lipoic acid to diabetic mice prevented the increase in cholesterol, atherosclerotic lesions, and health deterioration that the disease would otherwise cause. Diabetic mice that did not receive alpha lipoic acid began to show signs of lethargy and illness after three months. However, all of the diabetic mice that received alpha lipoic acid stayed healthy throughout the study period.

The authors wrote, "Remarkably, alpha lipoic acid completely prevented the increase in plasma total cholesterol, atherosclerotic lesions, and the general deterioration of health caused by diabetes." [18]

Other research showed that glutathione levels decline in the aging heart and brain. Treatment with alpha lipoic acid restored glutathione levels in the brain and improved age-related changes in both heart and brain tissue. The researchers concluded that alpha lipoic acid is an effective agent to restore the age-associated decline in glutathione. [19]

ALPHA LIPOIC ACID PREVENTS CATARACTS

Cataracts are the result of too much oxidative damage to the eyes after many years of exposure to the sun, pollution, and other toxins. Dr. Packer dramatically showed the difference alpha lipoic acid can make. In an experiment, he gave two groups of newborn rats a chemical that suppressed glutathione. He gave one of the groups an injection of alpha lipoic acid. At six weeks of age when the rats opened their eyes, the group that did not receive the alpha lipoic acid all had cataracts. Almost all of the rats in the alpha lipoic acid group had no cataracts! [20]

ALPHA LIPOIC ACID PREVENTS DAMAGE DUE TO STROKE AND HEART ATTACK

One danger in strokes and heart attacks is the lack of oxygen caused by the blood clot in the brain or the heart, leading to an initial process called ischemia. That's dangerous, it's true. But another danger can occur when the blood starts flowing again and the oxygen is restored. This is called reperfusion. The entire process of the blood and oxygen supply being shut down and then suddenly restored is called ischemia-reperfusion. When the blood and oxygen are restored there is an explosion of free radical damage, which overwhelms the body's natural antioxidant defenses, causing a tremendous amount of damage to the brain and heart.

Giving powerful antioxidants right after a stroke or heart attack appears to help protect against the massive free radical damage. In an animal study, it was found that giving alpha lipoic acid to rats protected them against stroke-related brain injury by boosting glutathione. In the non-alpha lipoic acid animals, glutathione had dramatically fallen after an induced stroke, indicating that the antioxidant defense against free radicals was put out of commission. These animals had clear-cut brain damage. The alpha lipoic acid treated animals had high levels of glutathione and were perfectly normal with no brain damage.[21] A similar experiment was done with the heart in animals. Alpha lipoic acid was added to the reperfusion solution and the recovery rate of the animals receiving the alpha lipoic acid was more than double the rate of recovery of those without it.[22]

Alpha lipoic acid also reduces the inflammation associated with atherosclerosis. There is now widespread agreement that atherosclerosis is a chronic inflammatory disease. Alpha lipoic acid helps reduce the inflammatory response, prevent damage to arteries that leads to lesions, and helps reduce the amount of bad cholesterol that sticks to arteries.[23] Slowly, the medical and scientific communities are realizing that all the chronic diseases (including heart disease, diabetes and Alzheimer's) and cancer have the root causes of inflammation and oxidative stress. Find a way to prevent abnormal levels of inflammation and oxidative stress, especially in the mitochondria, and you have found a way to prevent the diseases of aging. The mitochondrial antioxidants combined with the right vitamins and minerals do just that. The "Universal Antioxidant"—alpha lipoic acid—is a critical part of the team that can keep you living a long and healthy life.

ALPHA LIPOIC ACID HELPS MEMORY AND THE BRAIN

Brain cells are loaded with mitochondria and need a lot of glutathione to reduce free radical oxidation and stay healthy. Not every antioxidant can pass the blood-brain barrier—but alpha lipoic acid can. It is one of the best brain antioxidants we have.

Researchers found that when they used radiation to increase stress in the brains of mice, memory and motor function got worse. However, when they gave mice alpha lipoic acid prior to radiation, the mice did not lose their memory and performed well on the motor activities tests. The study concluded that alpha lipoic acid is a potent neuroprotective antioxidant.[24] [25]

LIVE LONGER AND LIVE BETTER WITH ALPHA LIPOIC ACID

At a conference held at the Linus Pauling Institute at Oregon State University in May, 2007, Dr. Tory Hagen discussed the current status of alpha lipoic acid. He concluded that in both animal and human studies, this compound has been shown to slow the aging process, improve blood flow in diabetics, detoxify the liver, enhance immune function and promote healthy blood sugar and many other functions.

Hagen commented, "Our studies have shown that mice supplemented with lipoic acid...aren't just living longer, they're living better—and that's the goal we're after." It's all happening in the mitochondria.[26]

ACETYL L-CARNITINE—THE FUEL SUPPLIER FOR THE MITOCHONDRIA

As we have seen, with antioxidants it's the team effort that counts. Hagen and Ames' research showed that acetyl L-carnitine (this is the most bioavailable form to take as a supplement) helped rejuvenate aging mice, but had a higher oxidation effect. What was happening? Acetyl L-carnitine supplied fuel to the mitochondria, which created more energy and younger acting rats. However, since burning fuel also creates a few more oxidants, it would make sense that increasing the burning of fuel by acetyl L-carnitine would slightly increase oxidation. That's what happened. Adding the mitochondrial antioxidant alpha lipoic acid to acetyl L-carnitine rejuvenated the rats *and* kept their mitochondrial oxidation low.

Acetyl L-carnitine is a fuel transporter for the mitochondria. Outside of the mitochondria is a special kind of fuel called fatty acids. By burning fatty acids, the mitochondria are able to make the energy we need to stay young and healthy. However, first the fatty acids have to get inside the mitochondria. They can't cross over by themselves. Fatty acids need carnitine to shuttle them across. Just think of lots of gasoline fuel sitting at a refinery. It takes tanker trucks to deliver that fuel to the gas stations so your car can fuel up. Just like a tanker truck, carnitine delivers fuel to the mitochondria. Carnitine does this over and over. It shuttles fatty acids into the mitochondria, drops them off, and even takes some cellular garbage back out. The mitochondria burn the fatty acids and create energy, the carnitine shuttles some more fatty acids in, drops them off, and the process repeats itself. Carnitine is the compound that already exists in the body. Acetyl L-carnitine is the supplement form of carnitine that is most effective.

FROM DIETARY AND STORED FATS TO FATTY ACIDS AND ONWARD TO THE MITOCHONDRIA

Fatty acids come from dietary fats and from fat stored in the cells or fat (adipose) tissue. If you eat a diet with higher amounts of glucose than the body needs for energy or storage of energy, your body makes fatty acids in the liver and stores fatty acids as triglycerides in fat tissue. When your body needs them, the stored triglycerides are released from the fat tissue as fatty acids. Fatty acids are a major fuel used for making ATP in the mitochondria—the main energy process in the body. Fatty acids are also important for the synthesis of other important molecules. Carnitine transports long chain fatty acids into the mitochondria.

ACETYL L-CARNITINE REVERSES AGING IN HEART MITOCHONDRIA

Scientists measured cell energy activity in the heart mitochondria of rats. The energy of older rats was about 40% less than younger rats. Treatment with acetyl L-carnitine reversed this condition and the heart rates of old rats were almost completely restored to the metabolic function of young control rats. Acetyl L-carnitine could be beneficial in treating congestive heart failure in humans.[27]

ACETYL L-CARNITINE PROTECTS BRAIN AND SPINAL CHORD MITOCHONDRIA AFTER STROKE

Aging causes brain mitochondria to function less efficiently. Having a good supply of fuel keeps brain mitochodria pumping out energy. Plus, as you age your chance of having multiple "ministrokes" or major strokes increases. Acetyl L-carnitine helps protect against damage that happens after mini- and major strokes. Acetyl L-carnitine helps protect the brain and the spinal chord from injury after a stroke or surgery that blocks blood flow.[28 29]

ACETYL L-CARNITINE PROTECTS AND REGENERATES NERVES IN DIABETIC PATIENTS

As we discussed above, damage to nerves, whether from diabetes or other causes, can be devastating. Acetyl L-carnitine has been used to help restore nerve function in diabetics and to increase nerve regeneration. Pain showed significant improvement in patients taking 1,000 mg daily. The authors concluded that the double-blind, placebo-controlled trials demonstrated that acetyl L-carnitine helped improve nerve fiber regeneration, vibration perception, and reduced pain in patients with established diabetic neuropathy.[30]

ACETYL L-CARNITINE FIGHTS CANCER FATIGUE, WASTING AND LOSS OF APPETITE IN HUMANS

Because it is needed to shuttle fuel into the mito-chondria, acetyl L-carnitine increases energy production in every cell in the body. This can be extremely important to patients who are fighting cancer. Cancer patients often have what is called "wasting" or cachexia where their muscle just deteriorates leaving them gaunt and exhausted. Often they have no appetite and lose weight. Two recent human trials showed that acetyl L-carnitine can help people with advanced cancer feel better.[31] Patients who were given oral doses of acetyl L-carnitine (the highest level was 3000 mg a day with no toxicity) had increased carnitine levels and their fatigue and sleeplessness improved and depression decreased. Their appetites and their lean body mass improved significantly. The higher doses showed the greatest results and the study showed that these higher doses were safe and caused no side effects.[32]

ACETYL L-CARNITINE IMPROVES FUNCTION IN HEART PATIENTS

As a cardiologist, I am seeing that the conventional practice of medicine does not have to be separated from the new alternatives. For example, acetyl L-carnitine improves heart function in angina patients when taken in conjunction with standard medication and reduces the death rate after heart attack in patients also given conventional treatment.[33] [34]

ACETYL L-CARNITINE HELPS RELIEVE DEPRESSION IN SENIORS AND ALZHEIMER'S SYMPTOMS

Acetyl L-carnitine helps relieve depression in seniors and has been shown to reduce some of the symptoms of Alzheimer patients.[35][36]

THE MITOCHONDRIA TEAM

Alpha lipoic acid and acetyl L-carnitine are two of the best friends your mitochondria can have. But they aren't the only ones. Vitamins C and E, coenzyme Q-10, and glutathione are all on the mitochondria team and are helped by these two friends. Plus, research is showing that resveratrol, quercetin and OPCs are an important part of the team, too.

6
RESVERATROL—SUPER ANTIOXIDANT FROM RED WINE PREVENTS CANCER, HEART DISEASE, DIABETES, ALZHEIMER'S, AND OLD AGE

Resveratrol has emerged as one of the most revolutionary and mysterious compounds in medical science. Resveratrol is most commonly found in red wine. It is a powerful antioxidant classified as a type of nonflavonoid polyphenol called a stilbene. It burst onto the scene with the French Paradox as one of the leading candidates in red wine responsible for the stunningly low rate of heart disease in France. Research on resveratrol exploded, resulting in over three thousand laboratory (in vitro) and animal studies showing that it was safe and that it had medical properties far beyond what was first thought.

RESVERATROL AND THE GOOD SIDE OF STRESS

Resveratrol is formed in grape plants in response to stressors in the environment like intense sunlight (UV radiation), drought, fungus, and infections. Resveratrol helps protect the plant so that it survives and thrives. Apparently, when animals or humans ingest resveratrol they benefit in a similar way—resveratrol protects the human and animal cells from the inflammation and oxidation that comes from stress so that the humans or animals can survive with better health. It's a gift from the plant world to us—all due to stress.

Resveratrol is primarily produced in grapes and is also present in lesser concentrations in other dark-colored fruits and berries such as mulberries and cranberries. For commercial purposes, it is usually extracted from the dried roots of *Polygonum cuspidatum*, known as Japanese knotweed. Because the environmental stressors that trigger resveratrol can vary from location to location and from year to year, the levels of resveratrol in wine grapes and other plants may vary. The use of pesticides, herbicides and irrigation can also affect the levels of resveratrol in red wine. So, simply drinking red wine or grape juice does not always provide a stable level of resveratrol. Resveratrol supplements that have been tested for potency are a more reliable source of predictable amounts. However, due to nature's genius in creating the synergy of all of the polyphenols in red wine, I recommend combining a supplement of pure resveratrol with a red wine extract that contains grape seeds and skins.

We know that quercetin works synergistically with resveratrol to keep it in circulation longer in the body.[1][2] The other polyphenols may have equally important synergies. A recent study by researchers at Tufts University using Concord grape juice reported that the combination of the polyphenols could decrease the effects of aging on the brain. "It may be that the whole is greater than the sum of its parts," lead author Barbara Shukitt-Hale wrote in the journal *Nutrition*.[3]

RESVERATROL—A POWERFUL MITOCHONDRIAL ANTIOXIDANT AND ANTI-INFLAMMATORY

If oxidation and inflammation are at the root of all chronic diseases, and if protecting the mitochondria from oxidation is the key to preventing cancer, heart disease, diabetes, Alzheimer's, and other chronic illness, then a compound that acts as a powerful mitochondrial antioxidant and anti-inflammatory would be incredibly valuable to modern medicine. Resveratrol does all this—and more.

Resveratrol has powerful antioxidant properties, especially in its ability to scavenge the really wicked superoxide free radicals and protect the mitochondria. This is probably due to its ability to increase nitric oxide. Resveratrol also helps maintain high concentrations of the super mitochondrial antioxidant glutathione, which scavenges oxygen free radicals.[4][5]

How antioxidant supplements actually work in the body is an area of controversy. Some antioxidants, like resveratrol, may not show up in high concentrations in blood tests. Some may be effective in laboratory in vitro tests, but ineffective in humans. Some may be effective in synergy with other antioxidants, but not when taken alone. However, scientists are now recognizing that the powerful effectiveness of resveratrol resides in its ability to trigger a variety of processes in the body, such as positive gene, hormone and enzyme reactions. Resveratrol also increases levels of nitric oxide and supports mitochondrial antioxidants like glutathione, and directly quenches free radicals.[6][7]

Resveratrol has primarily been known for its powerful antioxidant effects in scavenging free radicals. However, the latest research is showing that some of its most amazing medical benefits are in how it affects another powerful antioxidant, nitric oxide, and a certain enzyme called sirtuin. This enzyme may be the key to living longer, preventing diabetes and heart disease, increasing energy, endurance and mitochondria, and protecting against Alzheimer's and other brain diseases. Resveratrol is the only known compound that activates sirtuin.

Science is still discovering all of the exact mechanisms by which resveratrol works, however the results are clear. *Resveratrol protects the mitochondria from deadly oxidation* and protects the heart, brain, kidney and other vital organs from damage due to free radicals and inflammation. Resveratrol also reduces the oxidation of cholesterol and fats that cause damage to the arteries.[8] [9]

Resveratrol has been shown in laboratory studies to help

- Prevent aging
- Increase endurance
- Support health of mitochondria
- Reduce inflammation
- Prevent oxidation
- Reduce heart disease
- Limit damage from heart attacks and strokes (ischemia-reperfusion)
- Prevent diabetes
- Prevent cancer
- Protect against neurodegenerative diseases such as Alzheimer's
- Protect against osteoporosis
- Prevent skin damage from UV radiation
- Reduce effects of herpes

SAFE FOR HUMANS

Based on the successful laboratory and safety results over the last decade, resveratrol has been approved for trials with humans. There are now several human clinical trials in progress that are studying the use of resveratrol to prevent cancer of all types in healthy people and to treat colon and follicular lymphoma cancers; to investigate clinical dosages; and to examine the effect of resveratrol on cognition and memory in Alzheimer's patients.[10] [11] Clinical human trials are extraordinarily expensive and are usually only undertaken if they have the backing of a pharmaceutical company with deep pockets looking to develop a new drug, a nonprofit organization, a university, or the U.S. government. These resveratrol trials are sponsored by several universities and The Alzheimer's Foundation.

I certainly want to see more human clinical trials on resveratrol and gather more clinical information about its ability to reduce damage from heart attacks, prevent type 2 diabetes, heart disease and brain diseases. However, that may take years. Meanwhile, studies have shown that resveratrol has no harmful effects. Almost all of the research scientists who have studied resveratrol take it themselves, as I do.[12] However, because there are some unanswered questions about resveratrol's effect on some types of breast cancer, please check with your doctor before taking resveratrol if you have or have had breast cancer.

The lack of harmful side effects is a major benefit of resveratrol. As a doctor who must manage the side effects of many drugs, I find this is one of its most important properties. It does no harm.

THE RESVERATROL ANTI-AGING BOMBSHELL

Laboratory research on resveratrol during the last decade has been impressive, showing that it could protect against cancer, heart and brain diseases through its anti-oxidant and anti-inflammatory properties. This was impressive enough. However, resveratrol revolutionized medical history in November, 2006, with the publication of the anti-aging research of Dr. David Sinclair of Harvard University. What Dr. Sinclair and his team discovered is that resveratrol extended life span in obese mice and kept them healthy. Obese mice that ate a high-calorie diet of 60% fat and took resveratrol did not come down with diabetes, heart disease and other problems of obesity and aging—and they lived 24% longer (based on mice still alive August, 2007). Obese mice that *didn't* take resveratrol had more heart disease, diabetes and other diseases of aging and died earlier. *No other compound has ever been shown to extend life span and have such dramatic anti-aging effects.*

Dr. Sinclair had previously screened over 20,000 molecules to identify a natural plant molecule that could enhance the activity of a particular gene in vitro—*SIRT1*. (The sirtuin *gene* is indicated with italics; the sirtuin enzyme that is triggered by the gene is without italics.) The *SIRT1* gene is one of seven sirtuin genes. The *SIRT1* gene triggers the SIRT1 enzyme, which appears to have tremendous health benefits for humans. Resveratrol emerged from this screening as the winning candidate.

Why did Dr. Sinclair choose this one particular gene? There are seven sirtuin genes—why this one? The *SIRT1* gene and its enzyme regulate the production of insulin and glucose, the metabolism of fat, and the survival of cells. If a compound such as resveratrol could enhance the ability of this gene to improve all of these functions, it could help prevent many chronic illnesses.

Resveratrol did all of that and it did something else that made headlines all over the world. It mimicked the effects of caloric restriction (CR). Caloric restriction is the most effective known way to extend life span. However, as a clinical program it's just not practical. Most of you (including myself) will not reduce your calories by 40%—not even if it's proven to extend the number of years you live. Reducing calories by almost half, nearly a starvation diet, simply reduces the quality of life too much. So, scientists have been searching for a natural substance that would mimic the effects of caloric restriction without having to starve. They found it in resveratrol.

THE HARVARD STUDY—RESVERATROL EXTENDS LIFE, REDUCES DISEASES OF AGING

Dr. Sinclair had three groups of mice. The control group was fed a normal diet and maintained normal weight. The two other groups were fed a high-calorie diet (60% fat) and became obese. The only difference between the two obese groups was that one of the groups was also fed resveratrol. The results were astounding.

The high-calorie mice without resveratrol got fat and came down with all the common chronic illnesses of aging and obesity: type 2 diabetes, liver pathologies, high cholesterol and lipid levels, fatty lesions, inflammation, heart disease, and poor motor function.

The high-calorie mice with resveratrol got fat but did *not* have type 2 diabetes, heart disease, inflammation, or liver pathologies. They did have high cholesterol and lipids, but they didn't get heart disease. *Resveratrol also increased the number of mitochondria*, especially in the liver. Sinclair's scientists discovered that resveratrol prevented the bad side effects of a high-calorie diet in 144 out of 153 significantly altered pathways.

The mice on a high-calorie diet with resveratrol still got fat, but they stayed healthy and they lived 24% longer. Plus, the resveratrol mice steadily improved their balance and coordination as they aged. This is important because so many older people suffer falls and injuries due to lack of balance and coordination.

The effect of resveratrol on insulin was the most dramatic. It appears that resveratrol interacts with a specific protein enzyme, AMP-activated kinase (AMPK). AMPK promotes insulin sensitivity and increases energy metabolism. Type 2 diabetes is a disease of insulin resistance, so this discovery has profound implications for the prevention and treatment of type 2 diabetes. Increased energy metabolism, of course, comes from the mitochondria. *In plain English, what resveratrol did was turn on some special genes that regulate sugar and increased the number and health of the mitochondria.*

The authors of the Harvard study concluded that "resveratrol can alleviate the negative impact of a high-calorie diet on overall health and lifespan."[13]

THE FRENCH STUDY—RESVERATROL INCREASES MITOCHONDRIA AND ENDURANCE, AND REDUCES WEIGHT

At about the same time as the Harvard study, another remarkable study was done in France. In this study, mice given resveratrol ran twice as far as ordinary mice—plus the resveratrol mice had muscles super-charged with mitochondria and a reduced heart rate. They were physiologically just like athletes who had trained hard, but without the training. They even looked like trained athletes.

The resveratrol mice had muscles that were remodeled. In the words of the lead scientist quoted in *The New York Times*, "Resveratrol makes you look like a trained athlete without the training." [14] The mice were fed a high-calorie, high-fat diet like the Harvard mice, but they did not gain weight. They were given higher doses of resveratrol. The scientists say the mice did not gain weight because the resveratrol significantly increased the number of mitochondria in muscle cells. More mitochondria means the mice were able to burn more energy, burn more fat, avoid gaining weight, and keep their muscles sensitive to insulin. Once again, the key was how resveratrol affected the mitochondria.

How did resveratrol do it? Scientists think that resveratrol works by triggering a chain of events. First, resveratrol activates sirtuin, which activates PGC1-alpha, which stimulates cells to produce more mitochondria. PGC1-alpha generates more mitochondrial antioxidants as well. [15]

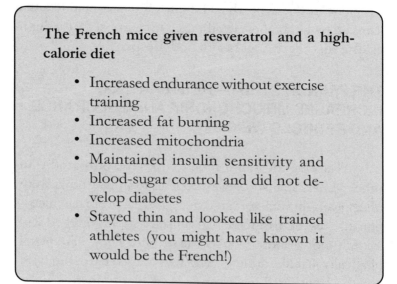

The French mice given resveratrol and a high-calorie diet

- Increased endurance without exercise training
- Increased fat burning
- Increased mitochondria
- Maintained insulin sensitivity and blood-sugar control and did not develop diabetes
- Stayed thin and looked like trained athletes (you might have known it would be the French!)

WILL IT WORK IN HUMANS?

These two studies are tantalizing. It worked in mice, but will resveratrol work the same in humans? The dosages were high in both studies. Translating dosages from mice to humans is not a one-to-one proposition. Scientists still have their work cut out for them to adapt these studies for humans. Dr. Sinclair and his lab are in the process of developing a drug to prevent diabetes based on the mice study. However, even though these experiments have not yet been proven to work the same for humans, there has been great interest in resveratrol in the business, scientific and medical communities. I do not recommend taking a massive amount of resveratrol because human and mouse metabolisms are not identical. Until scientists conduct human studies with relevant dosages, I will continue to take a moderate amount of resveratrol (100 mg of pure resveratrol plus a red wine extract) and recommend that you do, too.

The big picture of these studies is that resveratrol increases the number and health of mitochondria and helps control blood sugar levels and insulin sensitivity, reduces heart disease, and has a positive effect on endurance and coordination. Both studies confirm that in order to maintain energy, stamina, coordination, and health as we age, we must support our mitochondria and control oxidation with specific mitochondrial antioxidants.

RESVERATROL AND THE HEART

Heart research started the resveratrol revolution when Dr. Serge Renaud published a study to explain the French Paradox by showing that resveratrol inhibited platelet aggregation (blood clotting). Since then, much more research has revealed some astonishing effects of resveratrol on the heart.

RESVERATROL PRECONDITIONS AGAINST HEART ATTACKS

One of the most amazing new discoveries is that "resveratrol actually subjects the heart to a therapeutic amount of stress" that preconditions the heart against damage from a heart attack.[16] It appears to work the same way in protecting the brain, kidneys, ovaries, spine and the spinal chord from damage due to ischemia-reperfusion.

In order to understand this, let's review the term "ischemia-reperfusion." Ischemia-reperfusion describes what happens during a heart attack and stroke, or any time blood and oxygen are restricted and then restored. Ischemia is the restriction of oxygen by cutting off the blood supply. Reperfusion is the restoration of oxygen and blood. This sudden rush of blood and oxygen into the cells causes a tsunami of oxidation and devastating damage to the mitochondria. Imagine restricting a hose with water in it. The pressure builds up inside the hose and when it is finally released it shoots out with tremendous force that can cause damage.

WHAT IS PRECONDITIONING?

Scientists discovered that when they isolated animal hearts and subjected them to very low levels of restriction and restoration of oxygen and blood supply (ischemia and reperfusion) at regular intervals, and then subjected them to the level of a major heart attack, the prestressed, or "preconditioned" hearts experienced much less damage from the heart attack and the hearts recovered quicker. Preconditioning has been the "gold standard" of protecting hearts from damage due to a heart attack. According to one leading researcher, "preconditioning is the most powerful technique known to promote cardioprotection." [17] The problem is, it's not practical for people to show up regularly at their doctor's office to get their hearts stressed. And even if they did, this type of preconditioning doesn't last longer than a few days. It would be prohibitively expensive and inconvenient to implement as a preventive therapy. Therefore, the medical community has been looking for a drug or natural compound that would do the same thing. It appears that resveratrol does just that. [18]

Resveratrol reduces the damage caused by heart attacks in several ways. It increases nitric oxide that reduces mitochondrial oxidation, and increases expression of two chemicals (adenosine A1 and A3 receptors) shown to also be increased by preconditioning. It also activates the potassium channel. [19]

Isolated animal hearts with resveratrol that were subjected to ischemia-reperfusion heart attacks had improved ventricular functional recovery with better pressure and aortic flow, reduced myocardial infarct size, and reduced cell death due to apoptosis. *In layman's terms, it means that hearts that had been treated with resveratrol recovered in pretty good shape from what would have been a lethal heart attack.* Most researchers now think that although resveratrol works through several pathways, the most important are its ability to reduce oxidation damage to the mitochondria through the nitric oxide channel and to activate the potassium channel. [20] [21] [22]

As a cardiologist, I am very excited by the possibility that taking a supplement of resveratrol may help prevent the damage from heart attacks and improve the chances of surviving one. In the studies mentioned above, it was also found that a low concentration of resveratrol is optimum for the preconditioning of the heart, so it is very possible these results may be applied to humans. The regular consumption of grapes helped reduce damage from ischemia-reperfusion in an animal study.[23] According to one leading researcher, "There has been a desperate search for pharmaceutical preconditioning agents. Resveratrol appears to fulfill the definition of a pharmaceutical preconditioning compound."[24]

Certainly if you are at risk for a heart attack, or even if you are just getting older, taking a supplement of resveratrol is prudent. In any event, there's no harm in taking resveratrol in addition to any medications you are prescribed.

RESVERATROL PRECONDITIONS AGAINST PARALYSIS DUE TO VASCULAR SURGERY

In addition to protecting against the effects of a heart attack, resveratrol may help prevent one of the most dreaded complications of heart and lung surgery—paralysis. During aortic aneurysm repair surgery, the blood flow must be clamped off. A recent study at Columbia University in New York showed that pretreatment of rabbits with high-dose resveratrol reduced the incidence of paralysis after repair of thorco-abdominal aneurysms.[25] Again, the mechanism of action appears to be resveratrol's powerful antioxidant effect through nitric oxide promotion. Although more research on mechanism, optimal dose, and timing is needed, one group of researchers concluded that,

"...resveratrol may be used in humans as an adjunct to eliminate this catastrophic complication."[26]

RESVERATROL PRECONDITIONS AGAINST STROKE, KIDNEY, SPLEEN, ILEUM AND OVARIAN DAMAGE

Ischemic preconditioning has also been shown to protect the brain from the lack of oxygen that happens in strokes. In a recent in vitro study, resveratrol mimicked ischemic preconditioning via the SIRT1 pathway—the same sirtuin gene pathway that reduced aging in the Harvard mice and gave the French mice more energy.[27] A laboratory experiment with mice revealed that resveratrol has protective effects against acute ischemic stroke and that it may be a potential agent for the treatment of neuron injury in the brain associated with stroke.[28] Once again, the effect of resveratrol on the nitric oxide pathway appears to play an important role in protecting the brain.[29]

Other recent studies have shown resveratrol works the same way to protect the kidneys, ovaries, spleen and ileum from ischemic-reperfusion injury.[30 31 32] There is no downside to taking a moderate amount of resveratrol. Doing so may enable you to survive ischemic-reperfusion injury and prevent neurologic complications if you have to undergo vascular surgery.

RESVERATROL REDUCES LDL OXIDATION, INFLAMMATION, AND PROMOTES RELAXATION OF BLOOD VESSELS

Finding a way to reduce your risk of heart disease is one of the most critical steps you can take to live a longer and healthier life. Resveratrol addresses the two most important risk factors: oxidation and inflammation. The medical community has learned that it must consider the level of cholestrol *and* the oxidation of cholesterol. It is the oxidation of cholestrol that makes it dangerous. Resveratrol reduces oxidation of LDL (bad cholesterol) and helps reduce the formation of fat streaks in lesions along the arteries. Inflammation is the other risk factor that increases your chance of getting heart disease. It's important to know your level of inflammation as well as your level of cholesterol. Resveratrol reduces inflammation and helps prevent bad cholesterol and other fat molecules from sticking to arteries.[33]

Plus, as we have seen in the preconditioning studies above, resveratrol increases the supply of nitric oxide. Nitric oxide relaxes blood vessels, preventing rigidity that leads to high blood pressure. As blood vessels age, they lose almost half of their ability to relax. If lesions along the blood vessels exist, these restrict their ability even more. Resveratrol helps keep blood vessels relaxed so they can contract and relax normally, helping to maintain normal blood pressure levels. True to the promise of the French Paradox, resveratrol affects all of the factors in heart disease: inflammation, oxidation, blood clotting, relaxation of blood vessels, adherence of bad cholesterol to arteries, and increases your chance of surviving a heart attack.

RESVERATROL WORKS LIKE ASPIRIN—WITHOUT THE SIDE EFFECTS

Taking aspirin is a good anti-inflammation and anti-clotting preventive—except when it isn't. For many of my patients, a low-dose aspirin helps prevent blood clots and inflammation. I even recommend for my patients to take a regular size aspirin (325 mg), if it is not contraindicated for them, before going out where there will be a lot of sun exposure, such as the beach or the pool. When I take an aspirin with the resveratrol product that I use before I go out in the Florida sun, I find it gives me a much healthier tan color without the redness and sunburn and without having to use so much sunscreen. Using less sunscreen also increases my levels of beneficial vitamin D3.

However, for some people aspirin causes gastrointestinal bleeding, ulcers, and may be ineffective. Resveratrol could be a safe alternative. Resveratrol inhibits blood clotting by preventing platelets clumping together, just like aspirin. Resveratrol is a potent anti-inflammatory, just like aspirin. Some people are "aspirin-resistant," that is, aspirin fails to inhibit platelet aggregation. Resveratrol may work for them.

In a study of 50 high-risk cardiac patients taking at least 100 mg of daily aspirin it was found that 38% were aspirin resistant. Blood was drawn from the aspirin-resistant patients and resveratrol was added to the blood. Resveratrol significantly reduced aggregation, indicating that it could be effective in patients that aspirin didn't help.

Aspirin resistance increases with age. Only 26% of the patients in the study under age 60 were aspirin resistant while 45% of the patients over 60 were. The authors of this study concluded, "We propose that high-risk cardiovascular, aspirin-resistant patients will especially benefit from resveratrol consumption." [34] Resveratrol has been shown to have anti-inflammatory effects similar to the way in which aspirin works.[35] Although this was a laboratory study on resveratrol, I suggest that if you are someone who is aspirin resistant or you suspect you might have gastrointestinal damage from aspirin, talk to your doctor about using resveratrol.

RESVERATROL MAY PREVENT AND TREAT ALZHEIMER'S AND OTHER BRAIN DISEASES

In addition to helping the brain cells survive a stroke with minimal damage, resveratrol may be able to prevent and treat Alzheimer's. In fact, the probability of this, as shown in laboratory studies, is so great that The Alzheimer's Foundation has funded a human trial at Mt. Sinai Hospital to investigate if resveratrol can help memory and thinking in Alzheimer's disease patients. Alzheimer's is the most common brain disease. The Alzheimer's Association estimates that about 4.5 million Americans are already afflicted with this horrible disease and, if no cure is found, that number could reach 16 million in the next 50 years.

Alzheimer's disease is the accumulation of senile plaques in the region of the brain that controls memory. These plaques are composed of proteins called beta-amyloid peptides and cause a massive loss of neurons in the brain. Scientists believe that oxidative stress starts the breakdown of certain molecules that then form the damaging beta-amyloid plaques.[36] If there were something that could prevent either the oxidation or the formation of the plaques, it could prevent Alzheimer's. A third mechanism could also prevent Alzheimer's—the clearing of the plaques once they are formed.

Recent research on resveratrol and Alzheimer's found that resveratrol did not directly prevent the production of beta-amyloid plaques, but that *resveratrol did clear out beta-amyloid plaques that had already been produced.* This was a surprise and a huge breakthrough in Alzheimer's research. Resveratrol got rid of the dangerous plaques in the brain. The mechanism of action was believed to be that resveratrol triggered a kind of "clean-up" molecule called proteasome that targets proteins and gets rid of them. Resveratrol triggered the proteasome that cleared out the beta-amyloid protein in the plaques.[37]

Another study revealed that high levels of the SIRT1 enzyme provided powerful protection against the destruction of brain neurons by beta-amyloid plaques. Earlier, we discussed the Harvard and the French studies that showed resveratrol stimulated SIRT1 and reduced diseases of aging in obese mice and extended their lifespan. Now it appears that SIRT1 may play a role in the protection of brain cells. The researchers added resveratrol to their cell cultures and it strongly inhibited the toxic effects of the toxic plaques on brain cells. The authors of this study concluded, "Our findings highlight the potential therapeutic value of resveratrol and other sirtuin-activating compounds in protecting against neuronal loss in Alzheimer's Disease and related conditons."[38]

In research at the University of Paris, Christian Neri, research director of the Neuronal Cell Biology & Pathology Unit, discovered that resveratrol helped neurons resist the effects of Huntington's disease, another brain neurodegenerative disease. Again, the key was resveratrol's ability to activate sirtuins, which then triggered the cell's protective mechanism against the damaging Huntington protein. More research at Washington University discovered that resveratrol activated sirtuins that allowed cells to resist the degeneration that leads to multiple sclerosis, Lou Gehrig's disease, and Parkinson's. All of these are laboratory studies, but a clear pattern is emerging. Resveratrol stimulates sirtuin, a key enzyme that may prevent many types of brain disease.

Other studies have shown that giving red wine extract

that contained resveratrol to mice with beta-amyloid plaques slowed down memory loss and brain cell death. And it's not just the resveratrol in red wine that is helping. According to Dr. Sinclair of Harvard, quercetin allows resveratrol to circulate in the bloodstream longer and supports its benefits.[39] I am a strong supporter of taking a red wine extract and quercetin along with resveratrol for maximum benefit.

Resveratrol is the only compound known that stimulates this critical sirtuin gene that activates the SIRT1 enzyme that may help us live longer, have more energy, reduce diabetes and heart disease, and help us stay coordinated and functional—and now it may help protect our brain cells from the devastating destruction of beta-amyloid proteins that lead to Alzheimer's Disease. One of the leading resveratrol researchers, Dr. Leonard Guarante of MIT says, "It is now appearing that SIRT1 may be the universal regulator of aging. SIRT1 is expressed everywhere, in all tissues, including the brain."[40]

RESVERATROL MAKES MORE MITOCHONDRIA IN BRAIN CELLS

The Harvard study showed that resveratrol interacts with the AMPK enzyme to promote insulin sensitivity and increase mitochondrial energy. Another important study revealed that resveratrol activates AMPK in the brain, promoting growth of brain cells and increasing brain mitochondria.[41] As we have learned, the more brain cells and mitochondria, the healthier the brain will be, with enough energy to maintain cognition and memory. Pretty exciting stuff for one simple compound—resveratrol.

RESVERATROL MAY REDUCE RISK OF STROKE AND BRAIN TRAUMA

We discussed above how resveratrol may be able to precondition the brain to resist the damage to its cells from stroke. Now, researchers in Taiwan have discovered in a rat study that a single dose of resveratrol improved blood flow to the rats' brains by 30%, thereby reducing the risk of stroke.[42] Resveratrol probably stimulates the formation of nitric oxide, which increases blood flow in the brain and reduces the damage by stroke that cuts off blood supply. Other studies have shown that resveratrol protects against free radical-induced damage by restoring levels of glutathione.[43]

Brain injury and the resulting trauma have been making the headlines due to increased rates of brain trauma to soldiers serving in Iraq and Afghanistan. According to the Defense and Veterans Brain Injury Center, traumatic brain injuries afflict 14–20% of all military service members, and one in five vets of Iraq and Afghanistan. The high rate of brain trauma is believed to be caused by the striking of the head against the inside of the helmet when a roadside bomb explodes. If soldiers aren't screened, the trauma may be overlooked. Illinois is now screening all of its National Guard soldiers who serve in Iraq and Afghanistan for brain trauma.

What are the consequences of this type of injury? According to the *American Journal of Psychiatry*, March, 1999, the rate of psychiatric illness, including depression, is seven times higher in people who have had brain injuries. Panic disorder is more than 11 times higher. Resveratrol might be able to help. Researchers in Turkey who studied male rats found that treatment with resveratrol immediately after traumatic brain injury reduced oxidative damage and lesion volumes. The reseachers suggested that future studies with different doses are needed to determine the best dosage for humans. The dosages in this study were high.[44] Based on the ischemia-reperfusion studies with resveratrol that were effective at low doses, I think it possible that taking a moderate supplement of resveratrol daily might help prevent the oxidative damage that occurs with a sudden brain injury. It sure wouldn't hurt.

RESVERATROL REDUCES IRON IN BRAIN CELLS

Because we need iron as we are growing, we tend to think of having a lot of iron as a good thing. However, there is a growing amount of research that indicates that having too much iron, especially too much iron in our brain cells, is not a good thing. Some scientists believe that iron deposits in the aging brain mitochondria may be a significant cause of aging. Removing excess iron or preventing the accumulation of excess iron in the mitochondria may decrease chances of age-related brain diseases.[45]

Resveratrol may be able to accomplish this. In one study, resveratrol was able to cross the blood-brain barrier, reduce oxidation of fats, and increase the activity of protective antioxidant enzymes in the brain. The forms of most of these protective enzymes controlled iron, indicating resveratrol would be able to limit levels of free iron that causes cell and tissue damage in age-related brain diseases.[46]

Another experiment showed that resveratrol controls levels of iron in living tissue through its activation of the heme oxygenase enzyme. Resveratrol significantly increases this enzyme. Heme, a form of iron in the brain, damages cells by oxidation and this special enzyme breaks down this type of iron and helps protect brain cells. The researchers concluded, "Increased heme oxygenase activity by resveratrol is a unique way that resveratrol helps protect brain cells." [47] Resveratrol's ability to stimulate iron-protective enzymes could protect against stroke, amyo-

> **Resveratrol protects the brain in multiple ways:**
>
> - Reduces oxidation that causes damage to the brain mitochondria
> - Stabilizes cell membranes
> - Gets rid of amyloid-beta plaques that cause Alzheimer's
> - Stimulates sirtuin gene that protects brain neurons from damaging proteins
> - Activates an enzyme that promotes cell growth and increases mitochondria
> - Improves blood flow to the brain
> - Stimulates the formation of nitric oxide which protects brain cells
> - Reduces iron in brain cells

trophic lateral sclerosis (Lou Gehrig's Disease), Parkinson's, and Alzheimer's. Mice without this enzyme accumulate toxic amounts of iron in various organs. [48]

Some researchers believe that one of the mechanisms of action of caloric restriction in extending life may be the reduction of iron in the mitochondria of the brain. Maintaining cognitive faculties into old age may depend on your body's ability to clear excess minerals, especially iron, from brain tissue. Resveratrol appears to assist this process. [49]

How can you protect yourself against cancer?
Reduce inflammation and oxidation by taking a *combination* of natural antioxidants and natural anti-inflammatories that includes resveratrol and red wine extract, plus 1,000–2,000 IU daily of vitamin D3 and you may be able to reduce your risk of cancer by over 75%.

PROTECTION AGAINST CANCER

Here is some important information about reducing your risk of cancer:

- Chronic inflammation and the resulting oxidation is clearly correlated with increased risk of developing cancer.[50][51]
- Resveratrol reduces the development of cancer in all three pathways: initiation, progression and proliferation.[52]
- Resveratrol has potent anti-inflammation, antimutagenic and antioxidant properties.[53][54]
- Red wine drinkers reduced risk of colorectal cancer by almost 70%. The author of the study says the key difference between red and white wine may be that red wine contains large quantities of resveratrol.[55]
- Women who drink one or more glasses of wine per day have a 40% reduction in ovarian cancer.[56]
- Long-term consumption of more than one red wine drink per day resulted in 70% reduction in non-Hodgkin's lymphoma in men.[57]
- Red wine decreased incidence of prostate cancer by 50%.[58]

- A metabolized form of resveratrol (called a metabolite), piceatannol, may be one of the active anticancer agents.[59]
- Daily intake of red wine may prevent gastric cancer.[60]
- In a study of over 1,000 healthy, postmenopausal women, those taking 1,100 IU vitamin D3 plus calcium reduced cancer 77% compared to a control group.[61]
- Smokers taking a wide range of dietary antioxidants had up to 68% reduction in lung cancer. Researchers recommend smokers take a variety of antioxidants as a protection against cancer.[62] [63] [64] [65]

This is possible. You can do this. You can take resveratrol, red wine extract with 95% OPCs, alpha lipoic acid and quercetin. You can supplement with 1,100 IU of vitamin D3. Is it really that simple? I believe it is. Scientific studies provide convincing evidence that natural strategies work to reduce the risk of cancer.

Yes, it's also great to eat 5–15 servings of fruits and vegetables plus whole grains every day; cut out sugar, white flour, trans fats, junk food, hot dogs and lunch meat; exercise, lower stress, lose weight, stop smoking and reduce exposure to toxins.[66] *The problem is, the American population has been hearing this advice for years—and they still aren't doing it.*

Seventy-two percent of Americans eat only two servings of fruits and vegetables a day and one of them is potatoes. How many of you exercise regularly? How many of you can lower your stress? How many of you still drink a soda every day? How many of you still use commercial cosmetics, cleaning supplies, and bug spray? How many of you are overweight? *Simply telling people to do what has been proven they are not going to do is not going to reduce the risk of cancer.*

It's time to tell people another way to reduce their risk of cancer that they *will* do. I believe people will take a natural (or synthetic) substance that has no toxic side effects and will prevent cancer. Resveratrol is the leading candidate from plants.[67] Vitamin D3 is already a *proven* substance that prevents cancer based on a four-year, randomized intervention trial of postmenopausal women.[68] Yes, I also want you to make the lifestyle changes that will improve your health, but meanwhile, please consider taking the five supplements in this book, a multivitamin, and vitamin D3.

CANCER IS A HUGE PROBLEM

Cancer is such a big problem that my patients don't even want to think about it. They feel helpless. Somehow, they've gotten the idea that nothing can be done to prevent cancer so they don't even want to talk about it. Of course, dread of cancer is justified. It is the second biggest cause of death in the United States, and the number one cause of death for persons under age 85. One in two men will get cancer and one in three women. That's scary. Although immense amounts of money have been spent, thousands of researchers have published thousands of papers, and thousands of races for the cure have been run, overall incidence and mortality rates for all cancers combined have not changed much in 25 years.[69 70]

RESVERATROL INHIBITS ALL THREE PHASES OF CANCER

Even though a diagnosis of cancer is sudden and devastating, cancer is a disease that occurs over a period of 10–40 years. There is a continual process happening in your body in which cells are damaged that could lead to cancer. That's normal. Your body has several mechanisms to take care of those damaged cells. One is a strong immune system and another is healthy mitochondria that cause damaged cells to commit suicide (apoptosis) before the damage harms the DNA and the cell becomes cancerous. However, if you have elevated levels of inflammation and oxidation that weaken your immune system and your mitochondria as you age, you will have a lowered ability to fight cancer in all three phases.

A landmark study in 1997 demonstrated that resveratrol stops cancer in all three phases.[71]

The Three Phases of Cancer

1. Initiation—The Start of Cancer. Inflammation and oxidation damage mitochondria and cells.
2. Promotion—The Growth of Cancer. Cancer cells are not destroyed by the immune system or the mitochondria and they continue to replicate.
3. Progression—The Spread of Cancer. Blood vessel growth (angiogenesis) increases and feeds tumors; cancer cells mutate and spread throughout the body (metastasis).

How did scientists discover resveratrol as a cancer preventive agent? The story starts back in 1991, right around the same time as the French Paradox appeared on the news suggesting that red wine could prevent heart disease. The National Cancer Institute supported a program called "Natural Inhibitors of Carcinogenesis." Dr. John Pezzutto of Purdue University was one of the leading scientists in this program. The goal of the program was to find natural plant agents that could prevent cancer and had low or zero toxicity. They also wanted a compound that people could take orally, was affordable and not too weird (i.e., something that people would actually take). Over a period of five years, Dr. Pezzuto and his colleagues evaluated 166 active compounds from 32 plant species in the laboratory. Nine agents evaluated by the project were considered promising. Resveratrol emerged as the leader. According to Dr. Pezzuto, "One of the most fascinating molecules we have 'rediscovered' is resveratrol." [72]

When Dr. Pezzuto and his colleagues published their findings that resveratrol could stop cancer in all three phases, it caused a media sensation. It also triggered an avalanche of research into resveratrol as a cancer preventing agent that resulted in thousands of laboratory studies and several human clinical trials for cancer that are on-going as of 2007. [73]

Laboratory (in vitro) and animal studies found that resveratrol was able to prevent or treat the following cancers: [74]

- Prostate
- Breast
- Colon
- Esophageal
- Neuroblastoma
- Leukemia
- Skin
- Metastasis to bone
- Pancreas
- Lymphoma

- Ovarian
- Melanoma
- Liver
- Lung
- Stomach
- Oral
- Cervical
- Thyroid

Laboratory research during the last 15 years has confirmed that resveratrol is able to prevent or treat many types of cancer in all three stages. Resveratrol is nontoxic and doesn't harm normal cells. It can be taken orally as a supplement. The mechanisms of action are not completely understood, and won't be until human trials are completed, but some mechanisms have been proposed.

Proposed mechanisms of action of resveratrol[75 76]

- Scavenges free radicals and reduces oxidation
- Reduces inflammation
- Activates and deactivates critical enzymes, proteins, genes, hormones and chemicals
- Triggers cell death of cancer cells via the mitochondria (apoptosis)

Reducing your risk of cancer is no longer a mystery. Take a combination of supplements that includes alpha lipoic acid, resveratrol and quercetin, plus other polyphenols in a natural base such as a red wine extract with 95% OPCs. Scientists now recognize a whole food extract contributes natural synergies that are an important part of antioxidant protection. Take a daily multiantioxidant and anti-inflammatory supplement with 1,000–2,000 IU of vitamin D3 (cholecalciferol). You can do it. And to really complete your protection program, eat lots of organic fruits and vegetables (40% higher in antioxidants than nonorganic), stop smoking, lose weight, exercise, and reduce stress.

RESVERATROL INHIBITS HERPES

At least three studies show that topical resveratrol is effective against the herpes virus, types 1 and 2. The researchers discovered that in experiments with mice, a 19% resveratrol cream could prevent replication of the virus in female genitals. In one of the studies, resveratrol was tested against acyclovir, the most commonly used prescription antiviral, and resveratrol was equally effective.[77]

RESVERATROL MAY PREVENT OSTEOPOROSIS

Osteoporosis is the loss of bone strength due to lack of minerals such as calcium and vitamins such as vitamin D3. Both men and women suffer from osteoporosis, but bone loss is greatest in postmenopausal women, leading to the hunched back and danger of broken bones. Research revealed that lower levels of the hormone estrogen was linked to bone loss and doctors began giving many postmenopausal women hormone replacement therapy with estrogen. Unfortunately, this treatment increased the incidence of breast cancer so it has been discontinued. Now, it appears that resveratrol may be able to strengthen bones without the side effects of hormone replacement therapy. Resveratrol can activate the estrogen receptor but it does not appear to increase cancer formation.

Studies of cell cultures and animals showed that resveratrol had several ways of forming strong bones. Resveratrol turned on genes that form bones and turned off genes that destroyed bones. Bones got stronger with increased bone mineral and structure. Resveratrol was as effective as hormone replacement therapy, however it prevented the formation of tumors instead of increasing them.[78]

However, because resveratrol does appear to have some effect on estrogen receptors, if you are a breast cancer patient discuss taking resveratrol with your doctor.

THE MYSTERY OF RESVERATROL— BIOAVAILABILITY

One of the remaining mysteries of resveratrol is the puzzle of its bioavailability. This is one of the mysteries of resveratrol that will be investigated in at least one of the human clinical trials. Resveratrol is rapidly absorbed but then it is also rapidly metabolized in the duodenum and the liver so that its concentration in the blood is very low. Quercetin helps reduce the metabolism of resveratrol in the liver and increases its bioavailability. However, it is still puzzling how resveratrol exerts such powerful effects with such a low level in the blood.

Possible answers to this resveratrol puzzle

- The chemicals that exist after resveratrol is metabolized, called metabolites, could be the active compounds. Researchers in England found that a metabolite of resveratrol called piceatannol targets cancer cells and destroys them without harming normal cells. Piceatannol is produced within the tumor itself.[79]
- Unmetabolized resveratrol accumulates in the intestinal tract, the site of 70% of immune

cells in the body. It could be especially beneficial to the digestive tract (as in colon cancer)
or benefit the body by supporting the immune
system.[80]

- It only takes a tiny bit of resveratrol to make a
difference. Although high dosages of
resveratrol were required to prevent cancer in
cell studies, "exquisitely low daily doses" were
effective in preventing cancer in three rat
studies.[81]

- Animal studies have shown that resveratrol is
metabolized in the liver and excreted in the
bile, which enters back into the intestines to
be reabsorbed. This may also contribute to its
overall natural pharmacological activity.

THE TWO FORMS OF RESVERATROL AND THEIR STABILITY

There are two forms (isomers) of resveratrol, one
called "*trans*-resveratrol" and the other called "*cis*-resveratrol." Both of these forms can be attached to a
sugar molecule making two other forms as well, called
piceids. Almost all commercial supplements contain the
trans form of resveratrol.

At first, researchers thought only the *trans* form was
beneficial. Now, scientists are realizing that the *cis* form
may contribute benefits as well—especially by reducing
inflammation and oxidation.[82] The most recent research
states, "… the beneficial cardioprotective effects of consumption of foods and beverages containing resveratrol
(notably red wine) may thus be a result of the combined
effects of the two isomers."[83]

In solid forms like supplements, resveratrol exists predominantly as a *trans* form and is stable. In a liquid solution, like wine, both *trans* and *cis* exist, with some wines having higher amounts of *trans* and others having higher amounts of *cis*.[84]

Some companies that sell resveratrol have claimed that resveratrol is very unstable and must have special capsules or storage conditions. However, a very thorough study by leading resveratrol researcher, Milos Sovak, Ph.D., settled this question by investigating all the forms of resveratrol and concluding,

> ...we do not find any evidence to support the claims publicized in the popular media that resveratrol and/or its glycon are unstable when stored as solids under ambient conditions. Our data show that under normal storage conditions *trans*-resveratrol and *trans*-piceid are stable in excess of four years, well beyond the shelf life of most nutritional supplements.[85]

THE RESVERATROL REVOLUTION

The two researchers who led the Harvard longevity/obesity study summarize many of the benefits of resveratrol. Drs. Baur and Sinclair conclude,

> In mammals, there is growing evidence that resveratrol can prevent or delay the onset of cancer, heart disease, ischemic and chemically induced injuries, diabetes, pathological inflammation, and viral infection. These effects are observed despite extremely low bioavailability and rapid clearance from circulation...caloric restriction is probably the only other treatment for which such a broad

array of protective effects is observed in mammals. In addition, resveratrol treatment increases mitochondrial biogenesis [growth]…and, at least under certain conditions, improves insulin sensitivity.[86]

Resveratrol is also extremely promising as a topical and oral preventive of skin damage, wrinkling, and skin cancer. I cover that in more detail in Chapter 8.

Resveratrol is like no other molecule known to science. It is truly a medical revolution—a gift to humans from the humble grape.

7
RED WINE EXTRACT AND QUERCETIN—NATURAL ALLIES AGAINST HEART DISEASE, CANCER, LOW LIBIDO, AND INFLAMMATION

Wine is different. Throughout the ages, poets and philosophers have praised its virtues. I remember as a child hearing the phrase, "King of the Universe—Fruit of the Vine," which is said four times during the Passover Seder meal, and being intrigued by it. The English translation of this blessing, "Blessed are You, Lord our God, King of the universe, Who creates the fruit of the vine. (Amen)," made me wonder. Now, it seems that the ingredients of wine may indeed hold the key to human mortality and health, which would account for its ritual celebration in Judaism, Christianity, and in many other cultures. There are many proverbs and poems glorifying wine. Perhaps they were on to something.

> Drink a glass of wine after your soup, and you steal a ruble from the doctor.
> *Russian proverb*

> Wine was created from the beginning to make men joyful, and not to make men drunk. Wine

drunk with moderation is the joy of soul and the heart.
Ecclesiastes 31:35–36

Wine is at the head of all medicines; where wine is lacking, drugs are necessary.
The Talmud

There are more old wine drinkers than old doctors.
German Proverb

A man cannot make him laugh—but that's no marvel; he drinks no wine.
Shakespeare
Henry IV Part 2

Here with a loaf of bread beneath the bough, A flask of wine, a book of verse—and Thou.
The Rubiyaiyat of Omar Khayyam
translated by Edward Fitzgerald

In vino veritas. (In wine, truth.)
Pliny
Historia Naturalis

Wine is bottled poetry.
Robert Louis Stevenson

You rarely find these sentiments expressed about vodka, gin, or Diet Coke.

There is *something* about wine, especially red wine. Intrigued by the French Paradox that revealed Frenchmen who drink red wine have low levels of heart disease, scientists joined the poets and philosophers in seeking that elusive something. Researchers have conducted literally thousands of studies trying to identify *exactly* what is it about red wine that is so healthy.

Scientists have identified and investigated the individual components of red wine and discovered many benefits for the heart, the blood vessels and circulation, the brain, and almost every organ in the body. You can look at the chart below to see the many polyphenol components in red wine and red wine extract that scientists have identified. All of these polyphenols benefit your health. Population studies have shown that people who eat or drink higher levels of these kinds of polyphenols (resveratrol, OPCs, anthocyanins, quercetin, and catechins) have lower levels of heart disease, cancer, diabetes, osteoporosis, nerve diseases and all chronic diseases.[1] The strongest evidence of the health benefits of polyphenols, however, is in preventing and possibly reversing heart disease—just like the French Paradox predicted.

You already learned about the amazing benefits of resveratrol in the previous chapter. In this chapter, I'm going to discuss the incredible Nobel Prize-winning discovery of nitric oxide—and what red wine polyphenols have to do with it. I predict you are going to see much more about the connection between natural polyphenols like those found in red wine and how they contribute to nitric oxide and health in the coming years.[2] Taking a red wine extract that includes all of the components of red wine in a real food base, and not just the supplements of individual compounds, is important. Why? In a word, it's the *synergy*. Although I believe in adding individual supplements as needed to make a powerful health formula, I think it's also good to include a whole food extract whenever possible. Fortunately, red wine extract does have the

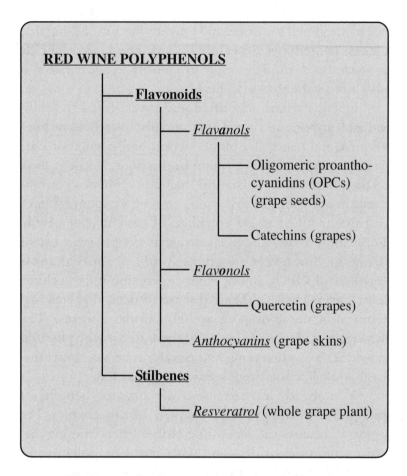

same effects as red wine—without the alcohol.

Scientists now believe that the health power of fruits, vegetables, and wine comes from the synergy of their components and in the ways you eat them together. A glass of red wine with a salad, olive oil dressing, and a steak is metabolized differently than a glass of red wine alone or just having a steak and potato. The olive oil helps prevent the harmful effects of the saturated fat in the steak and the red wine helps lower the oxidation levels that normally rise after you eat. Taking a red wine extract with

OPCs works differently than just taking a capsule of OPCs by itself. We may not know all of the ways that the components of red wine work together, but we know that they *do work*. People who drink red wine (or take an extract of red wine) have fewer heart attacks, lower blood pressure, fewer chronic diseases of all kinds, healthier circulation, nicer skin, may live longer and have a better sex life. And that's all part of the synergy and mystery of red wine.

RED WINE WORKS IN MORE WAYS THAN ONE

Since the French Paradox changed the course of heart research in 1991, thousands of studies have proven that the polyphenols in red wine improve the function of blood vessels, lower blood pressure, prevent blood clots from forming, lower inflammation in arteries, lower bad cholesterol and raise good cholesterol, prevent oxidation of bad cholesterol, and prevent damage to arteries that leads to plaque accumulation.[3] You already know about the antioxidant power of red wine polyphenols. Now scientists are realizing that polyphenols work in more ways than one.

The latest research says that red wine polyphenols may[4]

- Accumulate in *specific* tissues where they exert local antioxidant effects. This means that red wine polyphenols that have a specific affinity for an area of the body, may collect in that area. For example, scientists have known for some time that OPCs have a particular affinity for blood vessels and skin. They could be using their antioxidant power in these specific areas to prevent free radical damage.

- Produce low levels of antioxidants that turn up or turn down the signals between cells. Cells have to be told what to do sometimes. Research indicates that it only takes a low level of polyphenol antioxidants to act as signaling messengers.
- Regulate genes. Again, polyphenols may be the messengers that tell genes to do the right thing, not the wrong thing.
- Prevent the growth of blood vessels that feed a cancer tumor, thereby starving the tumor. Resveratrol, especially, has been shown to have potent anticancer effects, even at low levels.
- Break down into a metabolized form of antioxidants called metabolites. Scientists suspect that polyphenols that show low levels of antioxidants in the blood, like resveratrol and some of the other flavonoids, are broken down into active molecules that have not yet been identified. We know they work, but we don't always know how.
- Increase the activation of existing nitric oxide. The scientific evidence is very convincing that the connection between polyphenols and nitric oxide is critical to good health, especially heart health and a healthy libido.

That scientists do not yet know all the exact ways polyphenols keep us so healthy is not surprising. Research on polyphenols and how they prevent disease did not even start until the 1990s. Polyphenols and flavonoids were hardly mentioned in textbooks of medicine and nutrition before that. Your doctor may know very little about the health benefits of polyphenols if he or she was in medical school before 1995.[5] And considering that it can take years before doctors apply research into practice, the field of polyphenols is still very new. Antioxidants are one way that red wine polyphenols work. However, scientists have now identified other mechanisms of action as well.

"It is clear," said the author of a leading study of polyphenols, "that the mechanisms of action of polyphenols go beyond the modulation of oxidative stress."[6] In fact, the effect of red wine on the production of nitric oxide in your mitochondria could be the *most* important mechanism of all. Once again, it looks like all roads are leading to the mitochondria.

THE MEDICAL MIRACLE OF NITRIC OXIDE, THE HEART, AND THE MITOCHONDRIA

The discovery of nitric oxide (no, not nitrous oxide, the laughing gas) and how it helps your heart won the Nobel Prize in 1998. Dr. Louis Ignarro, Dr. Ferid Murad, and Dr. Robert Furchgott were awarded the Nobel Prize in Medicine for the discovery that nitric oxide was a crucial "signaling molecule in the cardiovascular system."[7]

It seems new ideas are always resisted at first. When Dr. Ignarro first presented his research in 1986 at a conference of prominent heart researchers at the Mayo Clinic, the reception was very skeptical. Major scientific journals rejected his papers. Eventually, however, the research was published showing that this very simple molecule of gas is produced within the body and helps keep our arteries flexible and relaxed, reducing plaque and lowering blood pressure. Finally, it was recognized that this insight into the workings of nitric oxide in the body was so important that he and two fellow researchers in nitric oxide were awarded the Nobel Prize in Medicine.

Nitric oxide does even more than help keep arteries flexible. It works with our immune cells to destroy bacteria and viruses. It helps the brain function and is also necessary for normal male erectile function and healthy female sexuality as well. *And, most importantly, nitric oxide has profound effects on the function of the mitochondria.*[8] Maintaining a healthy level of nitric oxide is absolutely critical to the balanced production of energy by the mitochondria. It's been shown that nitric oxide can even help the body generate additional mitochondria.[9] That's very important because as we age we lose mitochondria and our energy levels go down. Scientists eventually discovered that nitric oxide doesn't just lower blood pressure and reduce heart attacks, it influences the healthy functioning of every cell in the entire body.

Nitric Oxide[10][11]

- Supports production of energy in the mitochondria
- Supports healthy functioning of the entire cardiovascular system
- Reduces inflammation and formation of plaque
- Reduces oxidation in the mitochondria
- Reduces oxidation of cholesterol
- Helps white blood cells fight off invading bacteria, fungi and parasites
- Defends against tumors by triggering the death of damaged cells (apoptosis)
- Helps normalize blood clotting and reduces danger of stroke

THE IMPORTANCE OF THE ENDOTHELIAL LINING

Nitric oxide was discovered through its effects on the endothelial lining of veins and arteries. The endothelium separates the blood that flows through blood vessels—arteries, veins and capillaries—from the smooth muscles of the wall of blood vessel. When your endothelium is healthy, it is flexible and smooth and produces nitric oxide that keeps blood flowing and prevents unhealthy inflammation and plaque. Nitric oxide also helps fight off infection in the blood vessels. When high levels of insulin, inflammation and oxidation damage the endothelium, it becomes sticky like Velcro and stiff. It no longer makes enough nitric oxide and the damage just gets worse. More cholesterol gets oxidized causing more inflammation; high inflammation causes plaque to build up and then break off; and the tearing away of plaque causes blood clots that can cause strokes or heart attacks. Stiff arteries lead to high blood pressure and lack of circulation. All because the endothelial lining didn't get enough nitric oxide.

An unhealthy cardiovascular system, as we noted in earlier chapters, is the number one threat to a long and healthy life. If all types of cardiovascular disease were ended, Americans would live an average of nearly seven years longer.[12] If you maintain healthy levels of nitric oxide, you increase your chances of a having healthier mitochondria, a healthier cardiovascular system and a longer life.

WHAT'S WINE GOT TO DO WITH IT?

Obviously, having healthy levels of nitric oxide is critically important to preventing heart disease and producing mitochondrial energy. How can we increase our levels of good nitric oxide? Scientists now believe that having a diet high in flavonoid and nonflavonoid polyphenols like those found in red wine is one of the best ways to increase your levels of nitric oxide.

RED WINE EXTRACT GENERATES NITRIC OXIDE

Studies have shown that red wine extract generates nitric oxide, protects the heart, and promotes healthy sexual function. Red wine polyphenols strongly increase nitric oxide synthase, the enzyme reaction that helps produce healthy amounts of nitric oxide.[13]

A recent study showed that after three weeks of taking a red wine extract, blood pressure decreased in rats with high blood pressure that had low levels of nitric oxide. The red wine extract reversed the artery wall thickness, lowered blood pressure, and relaxed the arteries. All these effects of polyphenols prevent atherosclerotic plaque, the formation of blood clots, and strokes.[14][15] Another study with red wine extract showed that red wine enhances nitric oxide function and protects against metabolic syndrome, a cluster of cardiovascular risk factors.[16] Red wine contains unique polyphenol ingredients that increase nitric oxide and prevent endothelial dysfunction and subsequent atherosclerosis.[17]

As we noted earlier, *only half of all the people who have heart attacks have high cholesterol. The reason may be poorly functioning mitochondria.* Very recent research showed that low levels of nitric oxide result in poor mitochondrial metabolism that increases oxidation. This poor functioning of the mitochondria in the artery walls results in high blood pressure and atherosclerosis, but not high cholesterol.[18] Failure in the mitochondria due to aging and a reduced level of nitric oxide may be the root cause of atherosclerosis and heart disease. The polyphenols in red wine may be able to prevent that.

France and red wine have always been associated with romance. Maybe there's something to it. The research on nitric oxide established that erectile potency in men is dependent on having enough nitric oxide in the endothelial lining. The majority of cases of erectile dysfunction are associated with a damaged endothelial lining that cannot produce enough nitric oxide. Supplementing with high levels of polyphenols, antioxidants, alpha lipoic acid, and specific amino acids that naturally raise the nitric oxide level have been successful is restoring erectile function in many men and libido in women.[19]

RED WINE POLYPHENOLS PROTECT THE HEART

Studies on heart disease support the evidence that red wine extract high in flavonoids or purple grape juice protects the heart, especially by generating nitric oxide that protects the endothelial lining. Patients with coronary heart disease who drank purple grape juice improved their endothelial function.[20] A study of over 10,000 men and women showed that people with higher flavonoid/polyphenol intake in their diet had lower mortality from ischemic heart disease, lower lung cancer incidence, less asthma and reduced type 2 diabetes.[21]

A collection of population studies of more than 100,000 people have shown that the greater the intake of flavonoids from whole food sources, the lower the mortality from heart disease.[22] In one study, acute intake of red grape extract had a positive effect on the function of the endothelial lining in patients with coronary heart disease.[23]

Patients on hemodialysis frequently have heart

complications. A concentrated red grape juice taken for only three weeks improved lipoprotein profile, reduced inflammation, reduced oxidized LDL, increased good cholesterol, and significantly decreased LDL and Apo-B.[24] Grape polyphenols lowered key risk factors of inflammation, plasma triglycerides, LDL and Apo B in a study of postmenopausal women.[25]

There's something special about the synergy of nature, especially in red wine. Taking a good red wine extract preserves all the ingredients in nature's own recipe for keeping our hearts healthy.

QUERCETIN—A POTENT ANTI-INFLAMMATORY IN RED WINE

Quercetin is present in high concentrations in grapes, onions, and apples. It addresses both of the two root causes of diseases—oxidation and inflammation. It has potent anti-inflammatory and antioxidant effects and is also an excellent natural antihistamine. A friend related to me the story of a woman who was bitten by fire ants. She had a painful and immediate reaction similar to a bee sting. Although she took an over-the-counter (OTC) antihistamine, it didn't work. OTC antihistamines work by blocking receptors to histamine. Quercetin works by actually reducing the production of histamine. She knew that onions had a high level of quercetin, so she cooked up a big pan of onions and ate them and the swelling and pain immediately subsided.

Of all the polyphenols studied, quercetin had the most effect in protecting the endothelium from oxidation and cell death caused by apoptosis.[26] Quercetin is a good team player, too. It enhances the bioavailability of resveratrol and increases vitamin E levels in the blood and the liver. Vitamin E is a potent antioxidant needed by the body to fight free radicals. Taking quercetin may be more efficient than direct supplementation with vitamin E.[27]

Quercetin has an affinity for the liver and several studies have shown that it can support healthy liver function.[28] Its antioxidant power helps support detoxification in the liver.

Quercetin is good for the heart, too. A recent double-blind randomized study showed that people who ate soup with 69 mg of quercetin compared to soup with 5 mg of quercetin significantly reduced their risk of thrombosis and potential risk of heart disease.[29]

Therapeutic uses of quercetin* [30]
- Allergies, asthma, hay fever and hives
- Antibacterial
- Protective against cancers
- Heart disease
- Diabetic complications
- Eye disorders
- Gout
- Brain disorders
- Osteoporosis
- Peptic ulcer
- Herpes

*Most research done in laboratory (in vitro) and animal studies.

GRAPE SEED EXTRACT—ADDED POLYPHENOL POWER

An important component of a good quality red wine extract is the seed. Grape seed is the highest edible source of OPCs. Researchers in London have identified OPCs as some of the most biologically active polyphenols in their protective effect on the endothelial cells. OPCs work by suppressing a peptide (ET-1) that constricts blood vessels. This allows the blood vessels to be more relaxed.

One study found that the traditional way of wine making that soaks the seeds in with the wine produces wine with a much higher OPC content. A study compared wines from southwest France and Sardinia that were made by the traditional method with other wines and found they had surprisingly higher levels of OPCs—five to ten times higher! Population studies have also identified these regions with the lowest rates of heart disease. And—they found that OPC raises nitric oxide levels in the endothelium.[31] Grape seed oil, however, is not a good source of this polyphenol.

Blood Pressure

Grape seed extract was also shown to lower blood pressure of patients with metabolic syndrome in the first human clinical trial to assess the effects of grape seed extract on people with a combination of high blood pressure, excess abdominal weight, high blood cholesterol and high blood sugar. Forty percent of American adults (50 million) have metabolic syndrome. After one month, grape seed extract dosages of 150 mg daily and 300 mg daily dropped the average systolic pressure by 12 mm and diastolic 8 mm. The 300 mg dosage also reduced levels of oxidized LDL cholesterol. According to the researchers,

"Generally the higher the oxidized LDL the greater the drop." There were no side effects reported. Researchers from the University of California, Davis, presented these results at the American Chemical Society meeting on March 26, 2006 at Atlanta, Georgia.

Oxidation After You Eat

Grape seed extract has also been shown to reduce the amount of oxidation after you eat, especially after a high fat meal. Supplementing with 300 mg of grape seed with meals lowers oxidative stress (or you could drink a glass of wine from Sardinia or southwest France high in natural OPCs).[32]

Skin Cancer

Grape seed OPCs promote an immune response that prevents the formation of tumors. Researchers from the University of Alabama reported that hairless mice supplemented with OPCs extracted from grape seed had 65% fewer skin tumors than mice not supplemented.[33] There are a growing number of studies suggesting that grape seed extracts may benefit skin from the inside. Other studies have shown that taking an oral supplement of OPCs reduced reddening of skin when exposed to radiation.[34] In the next chapter, I'll tell you more about the powerful effects of red wine polyphenols, including grape seed, in keeping your skin beautiful and healthy.

Grape Seed, the Mitochondria and Cancer

Grape seed extract significantly inhibited growth of colorectal tumors in mice with a 44% reduction in advanced colorectal tumors. The grape seed extract stopped the rapid growth of cancer cells by causing the cancer cells to self destruct (apoptosis). Cancer is rampant cell growth due to loss of the cell cycle within the mitochondria. Grape seed extract appears to help regenerate the normal mitochondrial apoptosis function.[35]

Grape Seed and Healthy Veins

As we mentioned earlier, OPCs in grape seed extract have been used to treat problems with veins and capillaries, as well as arteries. A double-blind, placebo-controlled study found that grape seed OPCs taken at a dose of 100 mg three times daily improved the major symptoms of venous insufficiency. Heaviness, swelling and leg discomfort improved over a period of one month with 75% of the participants improving substantially. Other trials have found grape seed more effective than the bioflavonoid diosmin and the herb horse chestnut for strengthening veins. OPCs have also been used to reduce swelling after surgery and to reduce the development of dangerous blood clots during air travel.[36]

GRAPE SKIN MAKES A DIFFERENCE

The rich, beautiful red, purple, and dark blue-colored skins of grapes are more than aesthetically pleasing. The colored skins of grapes and dark-colored berries contain a powerful polyphenol—anthocyanin. Anthocyanins are strongly anti-inflammatory and are powerful antioxidants. Studies have have shown that they have a positive effect on collagen and the nervous system. They protect large and small blood vessels from oxidative damage. This helps protect capillaries in the eyes and skin. Anthocyanins have also been shown to reduce allergic reactions. They help prevent the oxidation of LDL cholesterol and protect endothelial cells as well.[37]

RED WINE IS SPECIAL

It appears that the poets and philosophers were correct. There really is something special about red wine. It protects your heart, your source of vital energy—the mitochondria, your cells, every organ in your body, and even your love life. Most importantly, there is a synergy to the components of red wine. That's why it's important to take a complete red wine extract that includes the seed extract high in OPCs, the skin, and all the trace elements. Nature put all these components together and now science is discovering that nature was right. Part of the mystery of red wine is in the synergy of all its polyphenols—working together.

8
GREAT SKIN, STRONG MUSCLES, AND LOTS OF ENERGY

Health is important, but how we look as we age is important, too. How do we know someone is old or unhealthy? The first clue is usually the skin. If skin is leathery, wrinkled, dull, or has deep grooves and lines in it, we perceive the person as old. The person's energy level is important, too. Someone with vibrant energy, no matter how many wrinkles they have, is perceived as young. Muscle tone is an important part of a youthful appearance. Maintaining healthy muscles past 70 is a challenge. You'll learn the most advanced information we have at this time on how to prevent muscle loss as you age.

Moving with ease and flexibility is also important. Someone who creaks out of a chair and walks stiffly across the floor because every joint in their body aches appears old to others. I have been made aware of a woman in her late 80s who moves like a teenager. She started taking supplements plus doing interpretive dance and qigong in her early 80s and the difference five years later is amazing. She swoops and glides into a room and you simply cannot believe she is nearing 90.

Fortunately, all of the information that scientists have discovered about how to remain healthy as you age shows on the outside as well as the inside! The principles are the same. High levels of inflammation, oxidation, and damage to the mitochondria will damage your skin, make your hair turn gray, drain your energy, destroy your muscle fibers, and inflame your joints. Low levels of nitric oxide result in damaged arteries, slow circulation, and low levels of energy and potency. Many of the same remedies for reversing or slowing aging of your heart, brain, and cells apply to your skin, hair, muscles, and joints. Alpha lipoic acid, acetyl L-carnitine, resveratrol, quercetin, and the red wine polyphenols that fight free radical damage and inflammation help us feel good *and* look good!

KEEP YOUR MITOCHONDRIA HIGH AND YOUR OXIDATION LOW

It's hard to feel, look or act young when you have no energy. Energy is what makes our skin glow and our eyes sparkle. Energy is what helps us be interested in new things, go places, relate to people, and have fun in life. People without energy call it, "sick and tired of life." You've learned throughout this book that "all roads lead to the mitochondria." The mitochondria are the source of our energy and oxidation is their greatest threat.

MAINTAINING YOUTHFUL SKIN[1]

A doctor friend of mine who had many children as patients said that the most important thing she looked for in a diagnosis of the severity of an illness was the skin. Even if the child had a high fever, if the skin maintained a healthy tone, she wasn't worried. However, when she treated a child with no fever who had sickly looking skin, she *was* concerned.

The skin is the first thing we notice when we judge someone as "old." Wrinkles, lines and grooves, dullness and sagging skin define aging from the outside. Fortunately, the principles of anti-aging apply to skin as well as the heart and internal organs. It makes sense because the skin is an organ, too—the largest organ of the human body. Healthy blood vessels and capillaries are important to good looking, glowing skin. Your blood vessels bring oxygen and nutrients to the skin cells, keeping them vital. Broken capillaries are unattractive and they impede the circulation that keeps skin healthy. Good circulation helps flush out the toxins that can damage skin.

You learned in a previous chapter how important it is to maintain a healthy endothelial lining. If your arteries and blood vessels fill up with plaque and inflammatory debris they cannot deliver life-giving oxygen to the heart. If the heart isn't pumping strongly, blood doesn't reach the skin and it gets a gray, sickly look to it.

Skin is composed primarily of collagen that binds skin cells together. High levels of collagen keep skin smooth and flexible. When you frown or smile, collagen helps your skin return to its smooth state. However, as your skin loses collagen it becomes stiff and less flexible. When you don't have enough collagen, your skin is less able to "snap back" and you develop deep lines and grooves.

Wrinkles are caused by oxidative stress within the cell that creates inflammation. Oxidative stress also produces an enzyme called collagenase that digests or breaks down collagen, resulting in microscars that lead to wrinkles.

The greatest dangers to healthy glowing skin are the

same dangers in all chronic diseases—oxidation within the cell and inflammation. Dr. Nicholas Perricone, M.D., one of the leading skin specialists, says that when he was first researching the cause of skin damage and looked at aging skin and young skin under the microscope, only the aging skin had inflammation.

The biggest contributors to inflammation of the skin are
- Sun radiation
- High levels of dietary sugar
- Dietary trans fats
- Pollution
- Harsh chemicals from soaps and lotions
- Stress
- Sleep deprivation
- Dehydration

In addition to causing inflammation, dietary sugar also contributes to glycation. Glycation occurs when foods rapidly convert to sugar in the bloodstream and cause the protein in your tissue to undergo a chemical reaction. When that happens in your skin, the sugar molecules stick to the collagen fibers. As more glycation occurs, this causes more and more molecules to stick together, resulting in the loss of elasticity. Your skin begins to look and feel leathery and stiff instead of soft and smooth. The bond formed between the sugar and the collagen also generates free radicals leading to inflammation and even more damage to skin cells.

Dietary trans fats are a cause of inflammation and damaged skin cells. Good fats like olive oil help the skin maintain its natural elasticity and glow.

RED WINE POLYPHENOLS PROTECT AGAINST SUN DAMAGE

Damage to the skin by UV radiation is activated after just five minutes in direct sunlight, triggering damaging free radicals in the cell plasma membrane. Although different types of skin react differently, all skin is damaged by the free radicals triggered by exposure to the sun. The assault of free radicals triggered by exposure to sunlight may eventually result in so much damage to the skin cells that they become cancerous.

Grape seed extract is one of your best allies in keeping your skin looking good. Several studies have shown that grape seed extract taken orally helps protect the skin. Researchers have concluded that the regular use of grape seed extract may help to protect skin from free-radical-mediated skin inflammation caused by sun exposure and to increase skin hydration.[2]

Another study showed that polyphenols at high levels reduced UV radiation damage 25% and improved skin texture, thickness and hydration. The mechanism of protection was believed to be that flavanols increase skin blood flow and protect against free radical damage. The study concluded that a beverage rich in polyphenols can confer substantial skin protection from the sun and help maintain healthy skin by improving skin structure and function. This study was done with cocoa, but would also apply to other polyphenol-rich foods and drinks like red wine, green tea, and red wine extract.[3] Other studies have confirmed that taking supplemental antioxidants, even at very low levels, protect the skin, keep it smooth, and prevent scaling as well.[4]

TOPICAL RESVERATROL PREVENTS SKIN CANCER!

According to the World Cancer Report, skin cancer represents 30% of all newly diagnosed cancers in the world and UVA and UVB radiation from the sun is an established cause of 90% of skin cancers. Current options have proven inadequate for the management of skin cancer and other adverse effects of UVA and UVB radiation. Sunburn prevalence is increasing in the United States. A study by the Centers for Disease Control showed that sunburn prevalence increased in all adults from 31.8% in 1999 to 33.7% in 2004, with men having a higher prevalence of sunburn than women in all three years with a shocking increase of 7% from 2003 to 2004 among men. In 2004, a total of 20 states reported increases in sunburns among whites. Utah had the highest prevalence of sunburn (51.3%) and Arizona had the lowest (25.7%).[5]

An important study published in 2005 investigated the use of topical resveratrol to prevent skin cancer. Researchers designed an experiment that exposed hairless mice to UV radiation while they were supplemented with resveratrol. They specifically designed an experiment that would most closely duplicate the human situation. This experiment clearly demonstrated that topical application of resveratrol resulted in a highly significant inhibition of tumor incidence.[6]

In this experiment, resveratrol imparted equal if not better protection if it was applied *after* exposure to ultraviolet radiation. So if you get a sunburn you can come home and apply resveratrol to minimize the damage. Resveratrol did not act like a sunscreen but was absorbed into the skin and activated a protective signaling cascade inside the cell that prevented the chain of events that leads to cancer. Resveratrol inhibited the malignant conversion of premalignant conditions such as actinic keratoses. Resveratrol appears to work by a sequence of events that kills off premalignant and malignant cells controlled by the mitochondria. Once again, we are seeing that all roads for health lead to the mitochondria—even keeping your skin healthy.

SUPPLEMENTS OF RESVERATROL AND OTHER WINE POLYPHENOLS

Resveratrol taken orally also protects the skin from damage that leads to skin cancer. Remember, the same kind of damage that causes cancer also causes your skin to become leathery and wrinkled. A review of 70 published studies in vitro and in vivo concluded that resveratrol treatment helped prevent damage to skin and stopped the development of cancer cells.[7]

A review published in 2006 cited several studies showing that resveratrol, quercetin, and grape seed extract triggered the process of apoptosis in the mitochondria that encourages damaged cells to commit suicide before they can mutate into cancer cells. This process doesn't affect normal cells. The review also noted that the protective effects of dietary agents such as resveratrol increase when combined with other dietary agents known to be cancer preventive.[8] Synergy is still the best strategy and is why a whole red wine extract supports single component supplementation. It might be wise to include an oral supplement of red wine extract, resveratrol and quercetin along with a topical application of resveratrol if you spend a lot of time outdoors.[9]

ALPHA LIPOIC ACID PROTECTS THE SKIN

Alpha lipoic acid is the universal antioxidant that can track down free radicals in the fat and water base of cells. It can penetrate into the mitochondria where most of the free radicals originate. While in the mitochondria, it also is part of the energy-producing system, making sure you have enough energy as you age. In Dr. Perricone's words, "...the higher the energy level in the cell, the more youthful you remain. The importance of alpha lipoic acid—the metabolic antioxidant—is hard to overstate." [10]

Alpha lipoic acid also inhibits a protein molecule called NF-kB that triggers inflammation chemicals called cytokines. Alpha lipoic acid inhibits NF-kB better than any other antioxidant. It blocks the inflammatory enzymes that damage collagen fibers so that your skin stays smooth and flexible. It also prevents glycation that makes collagen stiff and rigid.

Alpha lipoic acid affects the AP-1 factor. AP-1 is turned on by oxidative stress and digests your collagen leaving scars that turn into wrinkles. But when alpha lipoic acid turns on this enzyme, it only digests damaged collagen, not healthy collagen. It helps to remodel scar tissue—that's good!

Vitamins E and C are also vital antioxidants for the skin. As you have learned, alpha lipoic acid helps recycle these vitamins so they stay in the game of destroying free radicals.

Alpha lipoic acid also helps detoxify the liver by supporting healthy levels of glutathione. The liver is our primary detoxifer, but if it is sluggish and not working well then your skin will take up some of the load. As toxins are excreted through the skin they leave toxic residues that can irritate and damage the skin cells sometimes causing rashes. It's good to have a well-functioning liver so toxins are eliminated through the liver and the bowels and not the skin. Drinking a lot of water helps elimination through the bowels and will dilute toxins that come through the skin.

ACETYL L-CARNITINE DELIVERS FUEL FOR ENERGY

As we learned earlier, acetyl L-carnitine is necessary for the mitochondria to produce energy. It transports the right kind of fatty acids into the mitochondria for fuel, takes waste out of the mitochondria, and delivers more fuel. What a workhorse! Without enough acetyl L-carnitine your mitochondria won't be able to keep working and produce that beautiful energetic glow that lights up your skin. Taking a supplement of acetyl L-carnitine is an important part of a healthy skin program.

GRAPE SEED EXTRACT—A FRIEND TO THE SKIN

Grape seeds are high in OPCs that are known for having an affinity for the skin. They help support and stabilize collagen, protecting it from free radical damage and inflammation. As we age, our veins and capillaries become more fragile. OPCs strengthen capillaries and veins and maximize the delivery of oxygen and nutrients to our skin. OPCs help reduce inflammation and swelling after face lift surgery and help to prevent skin cancer.[11] OPCs from grape seed significantly inhibit the formation of proinflammatory cytokines such as nuclear factor kappa-B, which play a key role in skin damage from the sun.[12] Grape seed extract also stimulates the expression of a growth factor (VEGF), which is a crucial factor in repairing skin that has been damaged. Dosages ranged from 50–300 mg.[13]

NITRIC OXIDE RESCUES SKIN

You learned in the previous chapter that red wine polyphenols help generate nitric oxide. Nitric oxide also stimulates the synthesis of collagen and subsequent healing of wound sites and damage to the skin. Healthy levels of nitric oxide scavenge some of the most damaging free radicals. Nitric oxide keeps the endothelial lining of blood vessel healthy and is critically important to keeping your skin as well as your heart and your love life in good shape.[14]

QUERCETIN—FRIEND TO VITAMIN E AND A POTENT ANTI-INFLAMMATORY

Quercetin is a powerful anti-inflammatory and helps reduce the inflammatory reactions that damage collagen. Vitamin E is vital to skin health. Quercetin is also a powerful antioxidant and increases levels of vitamin E by attacking free radicals that reduce levels of this vitamin.[15] Quercetin also supports levels of glutathione in the liver and helps detoxification.[16]

GRAY AND THINNING HAIR AND ANTIOXIDANTS

Graying has always been associated with aging and sudden shock or trauma. According to an excellent study, the hair follicle is very susceptible to oxidative stress and high levels of stress can lead to premature graying. In fact, the graying hair follicle offers a model system to study oxidative stress and aging. By the age of 50, half of the hair follicles in 50% of all men have lost their pigment. Premature graying may serve as an indicator of biological response to a stressor. Mitochondrial DNA damage due to oxidative stress occurs in the follicles of graying hair. Mutations in mitochondrial DNA are caused by oxidative stress due to aging, inflammation and emotional stress.[17] There have been no studies to date using antioxidants to determine if they can slow down the graying of hair. It will be interesting to see the results! Meanwhile, I'll be doing my own experiment with alpha lipoic acid, resveratrol, quercetin, acetyl L-carnitine and red wine extract high in OPCs to find out for myself.

Thinning hair is also a marker of age and illness and OPCs have been shown to increase thickness of hair. In a Japanese study, researchers shaved the hair off mice and then applied a topical solution of OPCs to the skin. In mice without the OPC treatment, only 40% of their hair grew back. However, mice that had been treated with OPCs grew back 70-80% of their hair. Test tube studies confirmed that OPCs stimulate hair growth.[18]

MUSCLE AND THE MITOCHONDRIA

Muscle wasting is secondary to skin wrinkling as a marker of age. People appear old when their muscles are too shriveled and weak to give them the strength to walk strongly and gracefully. Sarcopenia is the medical term for the age-related loss of muscle mass, strength and functionality. It usually starts after age 40 and increases dramatically after the age of about 75. It can happen to people who are physically active as well as those who don't exercise. Scientists are just now beginning to address this serious problem. In addition to the loss of optimum functioning and the appearance of being old, the loss of muscle reduces the proteins and metabolites that help us survive trauma such as surgery and accidents. Aging muscle is no longer able to process proteins and sugars efficiently, and supplementing with dietary protein, carbohydrates and fats has not helped prevent muscle wasting. There has been some very encouraging research, however, using the amino acid leucine to prevent loss of muscle.[19] Sarcopenia has received much less attention than osteoporosis, though they are related conditions. Muscles generate the mechanical stress that keeps bones strong. When muscles are too weak to function well, it worsens the loss of bone.

The muscle that is connected to our bones consumes a large part of the body's total oxygen due to its large mass. When we exercise, it consumes the majority of the oxygen and produces the most free radicals. Skeletal muscle does not have the same capacity to repair its mitochondria that other tissue has, which accounts for the difficulty in preventing its deterioration as we age. Recent research measured the mitochondrial mutations in muscle fibers from aged rats and found much higher mutations in their mitochondria. Although it had been suspected that muscle loss was related to increased oxidative stress in the mitochondria, this is one of the first studies to prove it.[20]

In humans, aerobic exercise has not prevented loss of muscle mass. Repetitive weight training has had some effect, even in the very aged, but it is unlikely that most elderly people will engage in repetitive resistance training.

Vitamin E may help prevent muscle loss.[21] We know that carnitine plays an essential role in delivering fuel into the mitochondria and alpha lipoic acid reduces oxidative stress in the mitochondria, so supplementing with both of them has shown some success. In the experiment with aging rats by Dr. Ames and Dr. Hagen at the University of California, Berkeley, acetyl L-carnitine and alpha lipoic acid improved skeletal muscle. Alpha lipoic acid may also have the ability to restore the ability of skeletal muscle to absorb glucose necessary to normal functioning.[22] The latest research on mitochondria encourages me that there will soon be a solution to this difficult problem of aging. Supplementing with alpha lipoic acid, acetyl L-carnitine, quercetin (to support vitamin E), vitamin E, and an amino acid combination that contains leucine, plus repetitive exercise with weights, are the best strategies at this time to support healthy skeletal muscle.

I have noticed with my patients that those who look good also feel good. There is a psychological and a physiological mechanism at work. When you look in the mirror and you see a face full of energy with firm, healthy skin, shiny hair, and strong, firm muscles—you think of yourself as young. When you think young—you feel and act young. When your mitochondria are pumping out energy and your nitric oxide is repairing damage to your cardiovascular system and antioxidants and anti-inflammatories are protecting your collagen and your blood vessels are delivering oxygen and nutrients throughout your body—your smooth skin glows, your eyes sparkle, your muscles look fit and then you not only feel good, you look good, too.

9
YOU *CAN* CONQUER CANCER, HEART DISEASE, DIABETES, ALZHEIMER'S, AND AGING

As a medical doctor, I was surprised to find out how little I knew about the five super supplements in this book and their dramatic impact on heart disease, cancer, diabetes, Alzheimer's, and aging. It was a powerful insight for me to learn about the two root causes of all chronic disease—oxidation and inflammation. I was aware of the new research about inflammation and heart disease; I just had not read the additional research connecting it to the mitochondria, aging, and all chronic illnesses.

If you just look at the statistics, it is a gloomy picture. Diabetes has been declared a modern, world-wide plague and the incidence and death rate of cancer has hardly changed in 25 years. However, after learning about resveratrol, red wine polyphenols, quercetin, alpha lipoic acid and acetyl L-carnitine, I am very optimistic that we will stop these plagues in the very near future and live healthier and longer lives.

Because I am a practicing cardiologist and internist, I know that the medical procedures and medications I use daily save lives. I also am aware that surgeries and medications are expensive and may have life-threatening complications and unpleasant side effects. Even the cardiologist's friend, the humble aspirin, can cause side effects such as gastrointestinal bleeding.

I was not aware of these new super antioxidant break-throughs in chronic illness and aging until a few years ago. Like most doctors, I was not trained in medical school to know about red wine polyphenols and mitochondrial antioxidants. When I was in medical school, much of the research had not yet been done. Therefore, I was skeptical when I began looking into these supplements. Plus, like many practicing physicians, I work long hours seeing patients, making rounds, and keeping up with the major medical journals in my specialties. In order to learn about these new super antioxidants from red wine, plus alpha lipoic acid and acetyl L-carnitine, I spent many late nights on the Internet reading research papers.

I have written this book for you, and also for your doctor. I hope you share this information with him or her and discuss the advantages of beginning a super wellness and anti-aging supplement program. One of the great advantages of all these supplements is that they do no harm.

WHY SUPPLEMENTS?

One of my previous objections to supplements was my belief that you could get all the nutrition and antioxidants you need from a balanced diet. This, I now firmly believe, is not possible. There are three reasons why I believe you need to take supplements in order to sufficiently reduce oxidation and inflammation to maintain healthy mitochondria.

The three reasons I believe you need to take supplements

1. The recommended daily allowances (RDA) for nutrition set by the government are too low. These are really minimum levels that prevent overt pathology and disease. Dr. Bruce Ames, one of the world's leading researchers on reversing aging with alpha lipoic acid and acetyl L-carnitine, says our bodies need a full spectrum of micronutrients and that half the population may be deficient in at least one vital micronutrient. The simplest and most economical way to prevent deficiencies that may cause disease later in life is to take a supplement.[1]

2. The food we eat has dramatically lower nutrients than it used to have.[2] Shorter growing seasons, irrigation, and artificial fertilizers have increased yields needed to feed a growing population, but decreased antioxidants, minerals and vitamins significantly. For example, in a study published in the *British Food Journal* in 1997, all seven measurable nutrients in broccoli fell dramatically, notably calcium, which dropped 63% and iron, which dropped 34%. Over 25 fruits and vegetables had similar results. That means if we need to eat 5–10 servings of fruits and vegetables a day based on the previous nutrient values, we now need to eat 10–20 servings per person every day for the rest of our lives to obtain the needed antioxidants and nutrients. That is simply not possible for most people. Currently, 68% of adults do not even eat the minimum five portions a day.[3]

3. Modern lifestyles with high stress, poor sleep, toxins and junk-food diets create levels of oxidative stress that require higher levels of antioxidants and mitochondrial support than we can get from food. The super mitochondrial antioxidants such as alpha lipoic acid and resveratrol either are not reliably available from food or are better absorbed from supplements. Dosages of resveratrol vary greatly from wine region to wine region, depending on methods of agriculture and wine processing. Taking a supplement that has been tested for potency guarantees an effective dosage.

WHY WHOLE FOOD?

Although I strongly recommend taking the five super supplements in this book for an effective wellness and anti-aging program, I also believe you must have whole foods. A whole-food diet will include organic whole grains, nuts, fruits and vegetables, olive oil, pasture-raised beef or bison, free-range chicken and eggs, wild salmon and hormone-free dairy products. I wish all these were easy to find and economical. Unfortunately, this type of diet is just not possible for most people, including me. I do my best to eat well, but in my busy life, I simply cannot eat *perfectly*—and you may not be able to either.

In addition to a whole-food diet, I recommend whole-food extracts like red wine extract. Research shows that whole-food extracts deliver the same benefits as the food itself—however, they are usually more convenient and economical. Scientists are now discovering that there are trace elements and synergies in whole foods and whole food extracts that have benefits we cannot get from single compounds.[4] Nature created a wide range of compounds in natural foods. Scientists may not yet know what each trace compound does or how it works, but the growing consensus is that all of these elements *together* provide a synergistic matrix that maximizes the benefits of single compound supplements.[5]

I urge you and your doctor to review the information in this book carefully. By taking powerful supplements that support healthy mitochondria and reduce oxidation and inflammation, it is possible to dramatically reduce your risk of all chronic diseases. The next chapter provides a quick summary of the five supplements I recommend for living a longer and healthier life.

10
A QUICK GUIDE TO 5 SUPER SUPPLEMENTS

Because I know how long it took me to absorb and understand all of this new information, I have composed a quick guide for your convenience. It will make it easier for you to review why mitochondria are so important and to find the practical dosages and benefits for each of the five super supplements in this book. Please use it to refresh your own knowledge and to share with friends, family, and your family doctor. For more detailed information and references, please refer to the appropriate chapters. Pregnant and nursing women should consult their doctor before taking any supplements. These supplements are for adults. The dosages given are for maintaining daily health. If you are taking these supplements for a specific condition, please refer to the appropriate chapters and research papers for dosages and discuss taking the supplement with your doctor. In this guide, I list how each supplement works based on the most likely mechanisms of action reflected in the current research. Abstracts of scientific papers are available for free on the Internet at www.pubmed.gov.

MITOCHONDRIA

What are mitochondria?

They are tiny structures (organelles) inside almost every cell in our body that produce 95% of our energy. Mitochondria also destroy damaged cells before they can become cancerous.

Where are mitochondria?

Mitochondria are most abundant in high-energy organs like your brain, liver, heart and in skeletal muscle. *Each* cell in these organs and tissue will have thousands of mitochondria.

Why are mitochondria so important?

When mitochondria produce energy, they also produce most of the oxidation and free radicals in the body. To protect the mitochondria, there are mitochondrial antioxidants like alpha lipoic acid and glutathione. As you age, the amount of your mitochondria and antioxidants declines and free radicals increase. Free radicals damage the mitochondria and you lose vital energy and healthy function. Inflammation and age-related oxidative stress in the mitochondria are at the root of heart failure, cancer, diabetes, Alzheimer's, skin wrinkling, muscle loss, and aging.

How can we support healthy mitochondria as we age?

Eating a healthy, whole-food diet, exercising, and avoiding smoking and toxins reduces free radical damage to mitochondria. Taking mitochondrial antioxidants resveratrol, red wine extract with grape seeds and skin, alpha lipoic acid, and the powerful fuel provider acetyl L-carnitine supports healthy and abundant mitochondria.

How do these supplements support the mitochondria?
- Stimulate nitric oxide, a powerful mitochondrial antioxidant in the body
- Trigger important anti-aging genes and enzymes like sirtuin
- Reduce oxidation and inflammation
- Supply fuel to the mitochondria

SUPER SUPPLEMENT #1—RESVERATROL

What is resveratrol?

Resveratrol is a powerful natural antioxidant most commonly found in red wine, grapes and red wine extract. It is a nonflavonoid polyphenol that helps plants survive natural environmental stressors like fungi, drought, radiation and bacteria.

What does resveratrol do?

Resveratrol appears to transfer its ability to help plants survive stress to animals and humans who ingest it.

Can I get it from food?

Yes, resveratrol is present in grapes, red wine, dark grape juice, mulberries, and cranberries. Levels in food sources may vary greatly depending on growing and processing conditions. Commercial resveratrol usually comes from the root of the Japanese knotweed plant.

What are the benefits of resveratrol?*
- Protects the mitochondria from deadly oxidation
- Regulates sugar metabolism and protects against diabetes

- Increases the number and health of mitochondria
- Protects against damage from heart attacks and stroke by preconditioning the mitochondria
- May extend life span
- Reduces oxidation of LDL cholesterol
- Reduces blood clotting (platelet aggregation)
- Increases stamina and muscle
- Clears plaques that cause Alzheimer's
- Prevents cancer in all three phases
- Protects skin from UV damage and prevents skin cancer
- May prevent osteoporosis
- Inhibits herpes virus types 1 and 2

*Animal or laboratory (in vitro) studies.

How does resveratrol work?

- Stimulates nitric oxide that supports healthy blood vessels and reduces deadly oxidation in the mitochondria throughout the body
- Has the unique ability to trigger specific genes and enzymes that increase the number and health of the mitochondria
- Directly reduces free radical oxidation
- Reduces inflammation
- Triggers death of cancer cells

Daily Maintenance Dosage: 100 mg
Cautions: Breast cancer patients should discuss with their doctors before taking this supplement.

SUPER SUPPLEMENT #2—RED WINE EXTRACT

What is red wine extract?
A good red wine extract contains a high level (95%) of OPCs from grape seed, plus anthocyanins from grape skins, and natural amounts of resveratrol, quercetin, and catechins.

Is extract as good as red wine?
Yes. Studies have shown that red wine extract provides the same benefits as red wine.

What are the benefits of red wine or red wine extract?
- Lowers deaths from heart disease by almost 40%
- Reduces risk of colorectal cancer by almost 70%
- Reduces ovarian cancer in women by 40%
- Reduces non-Hodgkin's lymphoma in men by 70%
- Reduces blood clotting (platelet aggregation) and LDL oxidation*
- Generates nitric oxide that helps relax arteries and lower blood pressure
- Lowers blood pressure in patients with metabolic syndrome
- Lowers oxidation after meals
- Prevents skin damage
- Prevents skin cancer*
- Supports healthy veins and capillaries

*Animal or laboratory (in vitro) study.

How does red wine extract work?

- Stimulates nitric oxide, which protects the fragile endothelial lining in arteries, veins, and capillaries
- Reduces oxidation
- Reduces inflammation
- Promotes immune response that prevents formation of tumors

Daily Maintenance Dosage: 100 mg
Cautions: None

SUPER SUPPLEMENT #3—ALPHA LIPOIC ACID

What is alpha lipoic acid?

Alpha lipoic acid is a powerful antioxidant that protects the mitochondria. It is produced by every cell in the body. Known as the "Universal Antioxidant," it can penetrate into fat or watery parts of every cell. It also regenerates other antioxidants and can regenerate itself.

Can I get it from food?

No. Supplements are the best way to increase levels of alpha lipoic acid.

What are the benefits of alpha lipoic acid?

- Protects mitochondria from deadly oxidation
- Most effective known treatment for symptoms of diabetic neuropathy in humans
- Supplies fuel to the mitochondria to produce energy

- Saves liver from poisoning by regenerating the antioxidant glutathione
- Improves liver function in patients with hepatitis C
- Improves outcome in patients after myocardial infarction
- Reduces risk of cancer, heart disease, and other chronic diseases by supporting mitochondria health*
- Prevents increase in cholesterol and atherosclerosis*
- Prevents cataracts*
- Reduces inflammation in heart*
- Prevents damage from heart attacks and strokes*
- Helps memory and brain function*
- Slows aging*
- Enhances immune function*
- Promotes healthy blood sugar*

*Animal or laboratory (in vitro) study.

How does alpha lipoic acid work?
- Powerful antioxidant action protects mitochondria in all cells, tissues and organs
- Regenerates other antioxidants like glutathione
- Reduces inflammation
- Regulates important genes and enzymes

Daily Maintenance Dosage: 100 mg
Cautions: None

SUPER SUPPLEMENT #4—ACETYL L-CARNITINE

What is acetyl L-carnitine?

Carnitine is an amino acid in the body that supplies fuel to the mitochondria. Acetyl L-carnitine is considered the form most absorbable as a supplement.

Can I get it from food?

Yes. Lamb, beef and pork are the best dietary sources.

What are the benefits of acetyl L-carnitine?

- Increases energy by supplying fatty acids as fuel for the mitochondria*
- Reverses aging*
- Improves heart function in angina patients when taken in conjunction with standard medication
- Reduces death rate after heart attack, especially when given within 24 hours along with conventional treatment
- Significantly reduces pain and helps restore nerve function in diabetic patients
- Fights fatigue and wasting in cancer patients
- Relieves mild depression in seniors.
- May improve symptoms of Alzheimer's

*Animal or laboratory (in vitro) study.

How does it work?

Carnitine delivers fatty acid fuel to the mitochondria, which supports energy and healthy cells.

Daily Maintenance Dosage: 100 mg
Cautions: None

SUPER SUPPLEMENT #5—QUERCETIN

What is quercetin?
Quercetin is a powerful antioxidant, antihistamine, and anti-inflammatory flavonoid polyphenol.

Can I get it from food?
Yes. It is abundant in grapes, apples and onions.

What are the benefits of quercetin?
- Reduces inflammation
- Reduces allergies, asthma, hay fever and hives
- Protects blood vessels from oxidation
- Enhances bioavailability of resveratrol and vitamin E
- Supports healthy liver function
- Dietary quercetin may reduce risk of lung cancer
- May protect against prostate cancer*
- May also protect against diabetic complications, eye disorders, gout, osteoporosis, peptic ulcer, and herpes virus*

*Animal or laboratory (in vitro) study.

How does it work?
- Lowers inflammation and oxidation
- Lowers levels of histamine

Daily Maintenance Dosage: 100 mg
Cautions: None

References

Chapter 1

[1] Heart Disease and Stroke Statistics—2006 Update: A report from the American Heart Association Statistics Committee and Stroke Statistics Subcommittee. Circulation. 2006;113:85-151.

[2] Heart Disease and Stroke Statistics—2006 Update: A report from the American Heart Association Statistics Committee and Stroke Statistics Subcommittee. Circulation. 2006;113:85-151.

[3] Kritchevsky D. History of recommendations to the public about dietary fat. J Nutr. 1998;128(2):449S-452S.

[4] Kritchevsky D. History of recommendations to the public about dietary fat. J Nutr. 1998;128(2):449S-452S.

[5] The Wine Report. Available from: http://www.winesimple.com/featurelink1.htm.

[6] Marques-Vidal P, Arveiler D, et al. Patterns of alcohol consumption in middle-aged men from France and Northern Ireland. The PRIME Study. Eur J Clin Nutr. 2000;54:321-8.

[7] The Wine Report. Available from: http://www.winesimple.com.

[8] The Wine Report. Available from: http://www.winesimple.com/featurelink1.htm.

[9] Ferrieres J. The French paradox: lessons for other countries. Heart. 2004;90:107-11.

[10] Ferrieres J. The French paradox: lessons for other countries. Heart. 2004;90:107-11.

[11] Artaud-Wild SM, Connor SL, et al. Differences in coronary

mortality can be explained by differences in cholesterol and saturated fat intakes in 40 countries but not in France and Finland: A paradox. Circulation. 1993 Dec;88(6):2771-9.

[12] Marques-Vidal P, Arveiler D, et al. Patterns of alcohol consumption in middle-aged men from France and Northern Ireland. The PRIME Study. Eur J Clin Nutr. 2000;54:321-8.

[13] Ferrieres J. The French paradox: lessons for other countries. Heart. 2004;90:107-11.

[14] Renaud S, de Lorgeril M. Wine, alcohol, platelets, and the French Paradox for coronary heart disease. Lancet. 1992 Jun 20;339(8808):1523-6.

[15] Renaud S, de Lorgeril M. Wine, alcohol, platelets, and the French Paradox for coronary heart disease. Lancet. 1992 Jun 20;339(8808):1523-6.

[16] Blanco-Colio L, Valderrama M, et al. Red wine intake prevents nuclear factor kB activation in peripheral blood mononuclear cells of healthy volunteers during prostprandial lipidemia. Circulation. 2000;102(9):1020-26.

[17] Goldberg DM, Hahn SE, et al. Beyond alcohol: Beverage consumption and cardiovascular mortality. Clin Chim Acta. 1995 Jun 15;237(1-2):155-87.

[18] Opie L, Lecour S. The red wine hypothesis: from concepts to protective signaling molecules. Eur Heart J. Jul;28(14):1683-93. Epub 2007 Jun 7.

[19] Constant J. Alcohol, ischemic heart disease, and the French paradox. Clin Cardiol. 1997 May;20(5):430-4. Review.

[20] Goldberg DM, Yan J, et al. A global survey of trans-resveratrol concentrations in commercial wines. Am J Enol Vitic. 1995;46(2):159-65.

[21] Opie L, Lecour S. The red wine hypothesis: from concepts to protective signaling molecules. Eur Heart J. Jul;28(14):1683-93. Epub 2007 Jun 7.

[22] Wu JM, Wang ZR, et al. Mechanism of cardioprotection by resveratrol, a phenolic antioxidant present in red wine. Int J Mol Med. 2001 Jul;8(1):3-17.

[23] De Gaetano G, De Curtis A, et al. Antithrombotic effect of polyphenols in experimental models. Ann N Y Sci. 2002 May; 957:174-188.

[24] de Santi C, Pietrabissa A, et al. Sulfation of resveratrol, a natural product present in wine and its inhibition by natural flavonoids. Xenobiotica. 2000 Sep;30(9):857-66.

[25] de Santi , Pietrabissa A, et al. Glucuronidation of resveratrol, a natural product present in grape and wine, in the human liver. Xenobiotica. 2000 Nov;30(11):1047-54.

[26] Knekt P, Kumpulainen J, et al. Flavonoid intake and risk of chronic diseases. Am J Clin Nutr. 2002 Sep;76(3):560-8.

[27] Hayek T, Fuhrman B, et al. Reduced progression of atherosclerosis in apolipoprotein E-deficient mice following consumption of red wine, or its polyphenols quercetin or catechin, is associated with reduced susceptibility of LDL to oxidation and aggregation. Arterioscler Thromb Vasc Biol. 1997 Nov;17(11):2744-52.

[28] Opie L, Lecour S. The red wine hypothesis: from concepts to protective signaling molecules. Eur Heart J. 2007 Jul;28(14):1683-93. Epub 2007 Jun 7.

[29] Diebolt M, Bucher B, et al. Wine polyphenols decrease blood pressure, improve NO vasodilation and induce gene expression. Hypertension. Aug 2001;38:159-65.

[30] Nigdikar SV, Williams NR, et al. Consumption of red wine polyphenols reduces the susceptibility of low-density lipoproteins to oxidation in vivo. Am J Clin Nutr. 1998 Aug;68(2):258-65.

[31] Stein JH, Keevil JG, et al. Purple grape juice improves endothelial function and reduces the susceptibility of LDL cholesterol to oxidation in patients with coronary artery disease. Circulation. 1999 Sep 7:100(10):1050-5.

[32] Leikert JF, Rathel TR, et al. Red wine polyphenols enhance endothelial nitric oxide synthase expression and subsequent nitric oxide release from endothelial cells. Circulation. 2002 Sep 24;106:1614-7.

[33] Frankel EN, Kanner J, et al. Inhibition of oxidation of human low density lipoprotein by phenolic substances in red wine. Lancet. 1993 Feb 20;341:454-7.

[34] Hung LM, Chen JK, et al. Cardioprotective effect of resveratrol, a natural antioxidant derived from grapes. Cardiovasc Res. 2000 Aug 18;47:549-55.

[35] Hayek T, Fuhrman B, et al. Reduced progression of atherosclerosis in apolipoprotein E-deficient mice following consumption of red wine, or its polyphenols quercetin or catechin, is associated with reduced susceptibility of LDL to oxidation and aggregation. Arterioscler Thromb Vasc Biol. 1997 Nov;17(11):2744-52.

[36] Hooper L, Summerbell CD, et al. Reduced or modified dietary fat for preventing cardiovascular disease. Cochrane Database Syst Rev. 2001;(3):CD002137.

[37] Hu FB, Willet WC. Optimal diets for prevention of coronary heart disease. JAMA. 2002 Nov 27;288(20):2569-78.

[38] Kannel WB, Gordon T, eds. The Framingham Study: diet and regulation of serum cholesterol, Section 24. In The Framingham Study: An Epidemiological Investigation of Cardiovascular Disease. 1970. U.S. Government Printing Office, Washington, D.C.

[39] He K, Merchant A, et al. Dietary fat intake and risk of stroke in male US healthcare professionals: 14 year prospective cohort study. BMJ. 2003 Oct 4:327(7418):777-82.

[40] Kolata, G. Low-fat diet does not cut health risks, study finds. The New York Times. 2006 Feb 8.

[41] Howard BV, Van Horn L, et al. Low-fat dietary pattern and risk of cardiovascular disease: the women's health initiative randomized

controlled dietary modification trial. JAMA. 2006 Feb8;295(6):655-66. Available from: http://www.hsph.harvard.edu.nutritionsource/low_fat.html.

[42] Baur JA, Sinclair DA, et al. Resveratrol improves health and survival on a high-calorie diet. Nature. 2006 Nov 16:444(7117):337-42. Epub 2006 Nov 1.

[43] Mozaffarian D, Katan MB, et al. Trans fatty acids and cardiovascular disease. N Engl J Med. 2006 Apr 13;354(15):1601-13.

Chapter 2

[1] Associated Press. U.S. ranks 42nd in life expectancy. MSNBC.com. 2007 Aug 11.

[2] Anderson G, Horvath J. The growing burden of chronic disease in America. Association of Schools of Public Health, May 1, 2004, Public Health Reports, 119, 263-70.

[3] Anderson G, Horvath J. The growing burden of chronic disease in America. Association of Schools of Public Health, May 1, 2004, Public Health Reports, 119, 263-70.

[4] Rosamund W, Flegal K, et al. Heart disease and stroke statistics—2007 update: a report from the American Heart Association Statistics Committee and Stroke Statistics Committee. Circulation. 2007 Feb 6:115(5):e69-171. Epub 2006 Dec 28.

[5] Ford ES, Capewell S, et al. Explaining the decreases in U.S. deaths from coronary diseases 1980-2000. N Engl J Med. 2007 Jun 7;356(23):2388-98.

[6] Cordova AC, Sumpio BE, et al. The cardiovascular protective effect of red wine. J Am Coll Surg. 2005 Mar; 200(3):428-39.

[7] The Wine Market Council Report. 2002.

[8] American Heart Association; American Cancer Association; National Institute for NIDDK; National Heart, Lung and Blood Institute; National Coalition for Women with Heart Disease; Centers for Disease Control; American College of Cardiology.
Torpy JM, Lynm C, et al. Risk factors for heart disease. JAMA. 2003 Aug 20; 290(7):980.

[9] Renaud S, de Lorgeril M. Wine, alcohol, platelets, and the French Paradox for coronary heart disease. Lancet. 1992 Jun 20;339(8808):1523-6.

[10] Pignatelli P, Pulcinelli FM. Synergism among flavonoids inhibiting platelet aggregation and H2O2 production. Circulation. 2002 Feb 26;105(8):e53.

[11] Stef G, Csiszar A, et al. Resveratrol inhibits aggregation of platelets from high-risk cardiac patients with aspirin resistance. J Cardiovasc Pharmacol. 2006 Aug;48(2):1-5.

[12] Campbell CL, Smyth S, et al. Aspirin dose for the prevention of cardiovascular disease: a systematic review. JAMA. 2007 May 9;297(18):2018-24.

Chapter 3

[1] Shacter E, Weitzman SA. Chronic inflammation and cancer. Oncology. 2002 Feb;16(2):217-26.

[2] Ross, M. Chronic inflammation: rocking the medical world. Health Matters. 2004.

[3] Ross, M. Chronic inflammation: rocking the medical world. Health Matters. 2004.

[4] Bagchi D, Puri D. Free radicals and antioxidants in health and disease. East Mediterr Health J. 1998;4(2):350-360.

[5] Kregel K, Zhang H. An integrated view of oxidative stress in aging: basic mechanisms, functional effects, and pathological considerations. Am J Physiol Regul Integr Comp Physiol. 2007 Jan;292(1):R18-36. Epub 2006 Aug 17.

[6] Harman D. Aging: a theory based on free radical and radiation chemistry. J Gerontol. 1956;11:298-300.

[7] Van der Meide PH, Schellekens H. Cytokines and the immune response. Biotherapy. 1996;8(3-4):243-9.

[8] Kregel K, Zhang H. An integrated view of oxidative stress in aging: basic mechanisms, functional effects, and pathological considerations. Am J Physiol Regul Integr Comp Physiol. 2007 Jan;292(1):R18-36. Epub 2006 Aug 17.

[9] Kregel K, Zhang H. An integrated view of oxidative stress in aging: basic mechanisms, functional effects, and pathological considerations. Am J Physiol Regul Integr Comp Physiol. 2007 Jan;292(1):R18-36. Epub 2006 Aug 17.

[10] Greer EL, Brunet A. FOXO transcription factors at the interface between longevity and tumor suppression. Oncogene. 2005 Nov 14;24(50):7410-25.

[11] Ross, M. Chronic inflammation: rocking the medical world. Health Matters. 2004.

[12] Ridker PM, Cushman M, et al. Inflammation, aspirin, and the risk of cardiovascular disease in apparently healthy men. N Engl J Med. 1997 Apr 3;336(14):973-9.

[13] Ignarro L. NO more heart disease. 1st ed. New York: St. Martin's Press; 2005.

[14] Nissen SE. High-dose statins in acute coronary syndromes: not just lipid levels. JAMA. 2004 Sep 15;292(11):1365-7. Epub 2004 Aug 30.

[15] Chung HY, Sung B, et al. The molecular inflammatory process in aging. Antioxid Redox Signal. 2006 Mar-Apr;8(3-4):572-81.

[16] Lakatta EG, Levy D. Arterial and cardiac aging: major shareholders in cardiovascular disease enterprises: part II: the aging heart in health: links to heart disease. Circulation. 2003 Jan 21;107(2):346-54.

[17] Bejma J, Ramires P, et al. Free radical generation and oxidative stress with ageing and exercise: differential effects in the myocardium and liver. Acta Physiol Scand. 2000 Aug;169(4):343-51.

[18] Kregel K, Zhang H. An integrated view of oxidative stress in aging: basic mechanisms, functional effects, and pathological considerations. Am J Physiol Regul Integr Comp Physiol. 2007 Jan;292(1):R18-36. Epub 2006 Aug 17.

[19] Bakhru A, Erlinger TP. Smoking cessation and cardiovascular disease risk factors: results from the Third National Health and Nutrition Examination Survey. PLoS Med. 2005 Jun;2(6):e160. Epub 2005 Jun 28.

[20] Berkson, B. The alpha lipoic acid breakthrough. Paperback ed. New York: Three Rivers Press; 1998.

[21] Silver AE, Beske SD, et al. Overweight and obese humans demonstrate increased vascular endothelial NAD(P)H oxidase-p47(phox) expression and evidence of endothelial oxidative stress. Circulation. 2007 Feb 6;115(5):627-37. Epub 2007 Jan 22.

[22] Wellen KE, Hotamisligil GS. Inflammation, stress, and diabetes. J Clin Invest. 2005 May;115(5):1111-9.

[23] Baur JA, Sinclair DA, et al. Resveratrol improves health and survival on a high-calorie diet. Nature. 2006 Nov 16;444(7117):337-42. Epub 2006 Nov 1.

[24] Laufs U, Wassmann S, et al. Physical inactivity increases oxidative stress, endothelial dysfunction, and atherosclerosis. Arterioscler Thromb Vasc Biol. 2005 Apr;25(4):809-14. Epub 2005 Feb 3.

[25] Pace TW, Mletzko TC, et al. Increased stress-induced inflammatory responses in male patients with major depression and increased early life stress. Am J Psychiatry. 2006 Sep;163(9):1630-3.

[26] Knekt P, Kumpulainen J, et al. Flavonoid intake and risk of chronic

diseases. Am J Clin Nutr. 2002 Sep;76(3):560-8.

[27] Esposito K, Marfella R, et al. Effect of a mediterranean-style diet on endothelial dysfunction and markers of vascular inflammation in the metabolic syndrome: a randomized trial. JAMA. 2004 Sep 22;292(12):1440-6.

[28] Leighton F, Cuevas A, et al. Plasma polyphenols and antioxidants, oxidative DNA damage and endothelial function in a diet and wine intervention study in humans. Drugs Exp Clin Res. 1999;25(2-3):133-41.

[29] Urquiaga I, Leighton F. Plant polyphenol antioxidants and oxidative stress. Biol Res. 2000;33(2):55-64.

[30] Fitó M, Guxens M, et al. Effect of a traditional mediterranean diet on lipoprotein oxidation: a randomized controlled trial. Arch Internal Med. 2007 Jun 11;167(11):1195-203.

[31] Basu A, Devaraj S, et al. Dietary factors that promote or retard inflammation. Arterioscler Thromb Vasc Biol. 2006 May;26(5):995-1001. Epub 2006 Feb 16.

[32] Hodgson JM, Ward NC, et al. Increased lean red meat intake does not elevate markers of oxidative stress and inflammation in humans. J Nutr. 2007 Feb;137(2):363-7.

[33] Sies H, Stahl W, et al. Nutritional, dietary and postprandial oxidative stress. J Nutr. 2005 May;135(5):969-72.

[34] Han SN, Leka LS, et al. Effect of hydrogenated and saturated, relative to polyunsaturated, fat on immune and inflammatory responses of adults with moderate hypercholesterolemia. J Lipid Res. 2002 Mar;43(3):445-52.

[35] Liu S, Ridker P, et al. Relation between a diet with a high glycemic load and plasma concentrations of high-sensitivity C-reactive protein in middle-aged women. Am J Clin Nutr. 2002 Mar;75(3):492-8.

[36] Schulze M, Hu F, et al. Dietary pattern, inflammation, and incidence of type 2 diabetes in women. Am J Clin Nutr. 2005 Sep;82(3):675-84.

[37] Kitiyakara C, Chabrashvili T, et al. Salt intake, oxidative stress, and renal expression of NADPH oxidase and superoxide dismutase. Am Soc Nephrol 2003 Nov;14(11):2775-82.

[38] Rodriguez-Iturbe B, Vaziri ND. Salt-sensitive hypertension—update on novel findings. Nephrol Dial Transplant. 2007 Apr;22(4):992-5. Epub 2007 Jan 8.

[39] Wellen KE, Hotamisligil GS. Inflammation, stress, and diabetes. J. Clin Invest. 2005 May;115(5):1111-9.

[40] Berliner JA, Navab M, et al. Atherosclerosis: basic mechanisms. Oxidation, inflammation, and genetics. Circulation. 1995 May 1;91(9):2488-96.

[41] Sesso HD, Buring JE, et al. C-reactive protein and the risk of developing hypertension. JAMA. 2003 Dec 10;290(22):2945-2951.

[42] Ignarro L. NO more heart disease. 1st ed. New York: St. Martin's Press; 2005.

Chapter 4

[1] Harman D. Denham Harman and the history of the free radical theory of aging. Select Proceedings of the 2nd Annual Monaco Anti-Aging Conference. 2002 Aug 1;edited by Ward Dean. Available from: http://www.vrp.com.

[2] Wikipedia, Denham Harman. Available from: http://en.wikipedia.org/wiki/Denham_Harman.

[3] Lehninger AL. Water uptake and extrusion by mitochondria in relation to oxidative phosphorylation. Physiol Rev. 1962 Jul;42:467-517.

[4] Hagen TM. Oxidative stress, redox imbalance, and the aging process. Antioxid Redox Signal. 2003 Oct;5(5):503-6.

[5] Van Remmen H, Richardson, A. Oxidative damage to mitochondria and aging. Exp Gerontol. 2001 Jul;36(7):957-68.

[6] Linnane AW, Marzuki S, et al. Mitochondrial DNA mutations are an important contributor to aging and degenerative diseases. Lancet. 1989 Mar 25;1(8639):642-5.

[7] Linnane AW, Degli Esposti M, et al. The universality of bioenergetic disease and amelioration with redox therapy. Biochim Biophys Acta. 1995 May 24;1271(1):191-4.

[8] Garber K. Targeting mitochondria emerges as therapeutic strategy. J Natl Cancer Inst. 2005 Dec 21;97(24):1800-1.

[9] Bui T, Thompson CB. Cancer's sweet tooth. Cancer Cell, 2006 Jun;9(6):419-20.

[10] Bonnet S, Michelakis ED, et al. A mitochondria-K+ channel axis is suppressed in cancer and its normalization promotes apoptosis and inhibits cancer growth. Cancer Cell. 2007 Jan;11(1):37-51.

[11] Van Remmen H, Richardson A. Oxidative damage to mitochondria and aging. Exp Gerontol. 2001 Jul; 36(7):957-68.

[12] Navarro A, Boveris A. The mitochondrial energy transduction system and the aging process. Am J Physiol Cell Physiol. 2007 Feb;292(2):C670-86. Epub 2006 Oct 4.

[13] Bernal-Mizrachi C,Gates AC, et al. Vascular respiratory uncoupling increases blood pressure and atherosclerosis. Nature. 2005 May 26;435(7041):502-6.

[14] Nojiri H, Shimizu T, et al. Oxidative stress causes heart failure with impaired mitochondrial respiration. J Biol Chem. 2006 Nov 3;281(44):33789-801. Epub 2006 Sep 6.

[15] Chen Q, Camara AK, et al. Modulation of electron transport protects cardiac mitochondria and decreases myocardial injury during ischemia and reperfusion. Am J Physiol Cell Physiol. 2007 Jan;292(1):C137-47. Epub 2006 Sep 13.

[16] Hattori R, Otani H, et al. Pharmacological preconditioning with

resveratrol: role of nitric oxide. Am J Physiol Heart Circ Physiol. 2002 Jun;282(6):H1988-95.

[17] Adlam VJ, Harrison JC, et al. Targeting an antioxidant to mitochondria decreases cardiac ischemia-reperfusion injury. FASEB J. 2005 Jul;19(9):1088-95.

[18] Patil N, Chavan V, et al. Antioxidant status in patients with acute myocardial infarction. Indian J Clin Biochem. 2007;22(1):45-51.

[19] Peterson KF, Befroy D, et al. Mitochondrial dysfunction in the elderly: possible role in insulin resistance. Science. 2003 May 16;300(5622):1140-2.

[20] Santos MS, Santos DL, et al. Brain and liver mitochondria isolated from diabetic Goto-Kakizaki rats show different susceptibility to induced oxidative stress. Diabetes Metab Res Rev. 2001 May-Jun;17(3):223-30.

[21] Navarro A, Gomez C, et al. Vitamin E at high doses improves survival, neurological performance and brain mitochondrial function in aging male mice. Am J Physiol Regul Integr Comp Physiol. 2005 Nov;289:R1392-R1399.

[22] Gould E, McEwen, BS. Neuronal birth and death. Curr Opin Neurobiol. 1993 Oct;3(5):676-82.

[23] Hagen, TM, Ames BN, et al. Feeding acetyl-L-carnitine and lipoic acid to old rats significantly improves metabolic function while decreasing oxidative stress. Proc Natl Acad Sci U S A. 2002 Feb 19;99(4):1870-5.

Chapter 5

[1] Packer L, Colman C. The antioxidant miracle. Paperback ed. New York: John Wiley & Sons; 1999.

[2] Packer L, Colman C. The antioxidant miracle. Paperback ed. New

York: John Wiley & Sons; 1999.

[3] Packer L, Colman C. The antioxidant miracle. Paperback ed. New York: John Wiley & Sons; 1999.

[4] Khanna S, Atalay M, et al. Alpha-lipoic acid supplementation: tissue glutathione homeostasis at rest and after exercise. J Appl Physiol. 1999 Apr;86(4):1191-6.

[5] Berkson B. The alpha lipoic acid breakthrough. Paperback ed. New York: Three Rivers Press, Random House; 1998.

[6] Packer L, Colman C. The antioxidant miracle. Paperback ed. New York: John Wiley & Sons; 1999.

[7] Melhem A, Stern M, et al. Treatment of chronic hepatitis C virus infection via antioxidants: results of a phase I clinical trial. J Clin Gastroenterol. 2005 Sep;39(8):737-42.

[8] Hagen T, Ingersoll RT, et al. Acetyl-L-carnitine fed to old rats partially restores mitochondrial function and ambulatory activity. Proc Natl Acad Sci U S A. 1998 Aug 4;95(16):9562-6.

[9] Wright K. Free Radical: The eminent, controversial, and endlessly inventive biochemist Bruce Ames thinks he has found a way to slow the aging process in the brain. Discover. 2002 Oct.

[10] Hagen TM, Ames BN, et al. Feeding acetyl-L-carnitine and lipoic acid to old rats significantly improves metabolic function while decreasing oxidative stress. Proc Natl Acad Sci U S A. 2002 Feb 19;99(4):1870-5.

[11] Liu J, Atamna H, et al. Delaying brain mitochondrial decay and aging with mitochondrial antioxidants and metabolites. Ann N Y Acad Sci. 2002 Apr;959:133-66.

[12] Ames BN. Supplements and tuning up metabolism. J Nutr. Nov;134(11):3164S-3168S.

[13] Hagen T. Lipoic acid as an "anti-aging" and anti-inflammatory agent. Diet and Optimum Health Conference, Linus Pauling Institute,

Oregon State University, May 22, 2007.

[14] Ziegler D, Gries FA. Alpha-lipoic acid in the treatment of diabetic peripheral and cardiac autonomic neuropathy. Diabetes. 1997 Sep;46 Suppl 2:S62-6.

[15] Ziegler D, Nowak H, et al. Treatment of symptomatic diabetic polyneuropathy with the antioxidant alpha-lipoic acid: a meta-analysis. Diabet Med. 2004 Feb;21(2):114-21.

[16] Ziegler D, Ametov A, et al. Oral treatment with alpha-lipoic acid improves symptomatic diabetic polyneuropathy: the SYDNEY 2 trial. Diabetes Care. 2006 Nov;29(11):2365-70.

[17] Berkson B. The alpha lipoic acid breakthrough. Paperback ed. New York: Three Rivers Press, Random House; 1998.

[18] Yi X, Maeda N. Alpha-lipoic acid prevents the increase in atherosclerosis induced by diabetes in apolipoprotein E-deficient mice fed high-fat/low-cholesterol diet. Diabetes. 2006 Aug;55(8):2238-44.

[19] Suh JH, Wang H, et al. (R)-alpha-lipoic acid reverses the age-related loss in GSH redox status in post-mitotic tissues: evidence for increased cysteine requirement for GSH synthesis. Arch Biochem Biophys. 2004 Mar 1;423(1):126-35.

[20] Maitra I, Packer L, et al. Alpha-lipoic acid prevents buthionine sulfoximine-induced cataract formation in newborn rats. Free Radic Biol Med. 1995 Apr;18(4):823-9.

[21] Packer L, Colman C. The antioxidant miracle. Paperback ed. New York: John Wiley & Sons; 1999.

[22] Cao X, Phyllis JW. The free radical scavenger, alpha lipoic acid, protects against cerebral ischemia-reperfusion injury in gerbils. Free Radic Res. 1995 Oct;23:365-70.

[23] Zhang W. The role of lipoic acid in inflammation and atherosclerosis. Linus Pauling Institute Research Report. Available from: http://lpi.oregonstate.edu/ss03/lipoicacid.html.

[24] Manda K, Ueno M, et al. Radiation-induced cognitive dysfunction

and cerebellar oxidative stress in mice: protective effect of alpha-lipoic acid. Behav Brain Res. 2007 Feb 12;177(1):7-14. Epub 2006 Dec 4.

[25] Liu J, Atamna H, et al. Delaying brain mitochondrial decay and aging with mitochondrial antioxidants and metabolites. Ann N Y Acad Sci. 2002 Apr;959:133-66.

[26] Hagen T. Lipoic acid as an "anti-aging" and anti-inflammatory agent. Diet and Optimum Health Conference, Linus Pauling Institute, Oregon State University, May 22, 2007.

[27] Paradies G, Petrosillo G, et al. The effect of aging and acetyl-L-carnitine on the pyruvate transport and oxidation in rat heart mitochondria. FEBS Lett. 1999 Jul 9;454(3):207-9.

[28] Calvani M, Arrigoni-Martelli E. Attenuation by acetyl-L-carnitine of neurological damage and biochemical derangement following brain ischemia and reperfusion. Int J Tissue React. 1999;21(1):1-6.

[29] Postiglione A, Soricelli A, et al. Effect of acute administration of L-acetyl carnitine on cerebral blood flow in patients with chronic cerebral infarct. Pharmacol Res. 1991 Apr;23(3):241-6.

[30] Sima AA, Calvani M, et al. Acetyl L-carnitine improves pain, nerve regeneration, and vibratory perception in patients with chronic diabetic neuropathy: an analysis of two randomized placebo-controlled trials. Diabetes Care. 2005 Jan;28(1):89-94.

[31] Gramignano G, Lusso MR, et al. Efficacy of L-carnitine administration on fatigue, nutritional status, oxidative stress, and related quality of life in 12 advanced cancer patients undergoing anticancer therapy. Nutrition. 2006 Feb;22(2):136-45.

[32] Cruciani RA, Dvorkin E, et al. Safety, tolerability and symptom outcomes associated with L-carnitine supplementation in patients with cancer, fatigue, and carnitine deficiency: a phase I/II study. J Pain Symptom Manage. 2006 Dec:32(6):551-9.

[33] Singh RB, Niaz MA, et al. A randomized, double-blind, placebo-controlled trial of L-carnitine in suspectetd acute myocardial

infarction. Postgrad Med J. 1996 Jan;72(843):45-50.

[34] Davini P, Bigalli A, et al. Controlled study on L-carnitine therapeutic efficacy in post-infarction. Drugs Exp Clin Res. 1992;18(8):355-365.

[35] Garzya G, Corallo D, et al. Evaluation of the effects of L-acetyl carnitine on senile patients suffering from depression. Drugs Exp Clin Res. 1990;16:101-106

[36] Brooks JO 3d, Yesavage JA, et al. Acetyl-L-carnitine slows decline in younger patients with Alzheimer's disease: a reanalysis of a double-blind, placebo-controlled trial using the trilinear approach. Int Psychogeriatr. 1998; 10:193-203.

Chapter 6

[1] de Santi C, Pietrabissa A, et al. Sulphation of resveratrol, a natural product present in grapes and wine, in the human liver and duodenum. Xenobiotica. 2000 Jun;30(6):609-17.

[2] de Santi C, Pietrabissa A, et al. Glucuronidation of resveratrol, a natural product present in grape and wine, in the human liver. Xenobiotica. 2000 Nov;30(11):1047-54.

[3] Shukitt-Hale B, Joseph JA, et al. Effects of concord grape juice on cognitive and motor deficits in aging. Nutrition. 2006 Mar;22(3):295-302. Epub 2006 Jan 18.

[4] Miura T, Muraoka S, et al. Inactivation of creatine kinase induced by stilbene derivatives. Pharmacol Toxicol. 2002 Feb;90(2):66-72.

[5] Das DK, Maulik N. Resveratrol in cardioprotection: a therapeutic promise of alternative medicine. Mol Interv. 2006 Feb;6(1):36-47.

[6] Das DK, Maulik N. Resveratrol in cardioprotection: a therapeutic promise of alternative medicine. Mol Interv. 2006 Feb;6(1):36-47.

[7] Miura T, Muraoka S, et al. Inactivation of creatine kinase induced

by stilbene derivatives. Pharmacol Toxicol. 2002 Feb;90(2):66-72.

[8] Brito P, Almeida LM, et al. The interaction of resveratrol with ferrylmyoglobin and peroxynitrite; protection against LDL oxidation. Free Radic Res. 2002 Jun;36(6):621-31.

[9] Subbaramaiah K, Michaluart P, et al. Resveratrol inhibits cyclooxygenase-2 transcription in human mammary epithelial cells. Ann N Y Acad Sci. 1999;889:214-23.

[10] Clinical Trials.gov [homepage on the Internet]. U.S. National Institutes of Health, National Library of Medicine. Available from: http://www.clinicaltrials.gov.

[11] Mt. Sinai Medical Center [homepage on the Internet]. Mt. Sinai Alzheimer's Disease Research Center, Clinical Research. Dept of Psychiatry. Available from: http://www.mssm.edu/psychiatry/adrc/clinical_trials.shtml.

[12] Wade, N. Yes, red wine holds answer. Check dosage. The New York Times. 2006 Nov 2.

[13] Baur JA, Sinclair DA, et al. Resveratrol improves health and survival of mice on a high-calorie diet. Nature. 2006 Nov 16;444(7117):337-42. Epub 2006 Nov 1.

[14] Wade, N. Red wine ingredient increases endurance. The New York Times. 2006 Nov 17.

[15] Lagouge M, Auwerx J, et al. Resveratrol improves mitochondrial function and protects against metabolic disease by activating SIRT1 and PGC-1alpha. Cell. 2006 Dec 15;127(6):1109-22. Epub 2006 Nov 16.

[16] Das DK, Maulik N. Resveratrol in cardioprotection: a therapeutic promise of alternative medicine. Mol Interv. 2006 Feb;6(1):36-47.

[17] Das DK, Maulik N. Resveratrol in cardioprotection: a therapeutic promise of alternative medicine. Mol Interv. 2006 Feb;6(1):36-47.

[18] Das DK, Maulik N. Resveratrol in cardioprotection: a therapeutic promise of alternative medicine. Mol Interv. 2006 Feb;6(1):36-47.

[19] Hattori R, Das DK, et al. Pharmacological preconditioning with resveratrol: role of nitric oxide. Am J Physiol Heart Circ Physiol. 2002 Jun:282(6):H1988-95.

[20] Bradamante S, Barenghi L, et al. Resveratrol provides late-phase cardioprotection by means of a nitric oxide- and adenosine-mediated mechanism. Eur J Pharmacol. 2003 Mar 28;465(1-2):115-23.

[21] Imamura G, Bertelli A, et al. Pharmacological preconditioning with resveratrol: an insight with iNOS knockout mice. Am J Physiol Heart Circ Physiol. 2002 Jun;282(6):H1996-2003.

[22] Goh S, Woodman OL, et al. The red wine antioxidant resveratrol prevents cardiomyocyte injury following ischemia-reperfusion via multiple sites and mechanisms. Antioxid Redox Signal. 2007 Jan;9(1):101-13.

[23] Cui J, Das DK, et al. Reduction of myocardial ischemia reperfusion injury with regular consumption of grapes. Ann N Y Acad Sci. 2002 May:957:302-7.

[24] Das DK, Maulik N. Resveratrol in cardioprotection: a therapeutic promise of alternative medicine. Mol Interv. 2006 Feb;6(1):36-47.

[25] Kaplan S, Bisleri G, et al. Resveratrol, a natural red wine polyphenol, reduces ischemia-reperfusion-induced spinal cord injury. Ann Thorac Surg. 2005 Dec;80(6):2242-9.

[26] Kiziltepe U, Turan NN, et al. Resveratrol, a red wine polyphenol protects spinal cord from ischemia-reperfusion injury. J Vasc Surg. 2004 Jul; 40(1):138-45.

[27] Raval A, Cave KR, et al. Resveratrol mimics ischemic preconditioning in the brain. J Cereb Blood Flow Metab. 2006 Sep;26(9):1141-7. Epub 2005 Dec 14.

[28] Gao D, Zhang X, et al. Resveratrol reduces the elevated level of MMP-9 induced by cerebral ischemia-reperfusion in mice. Life Sci. 2006 Apr 25;78(22):2564-70.

[29] Tsai SK, Hung LM, et al. Resveratrol neuroprotective effects during focal cerebral ischemia injury via nitric oxide mechanism in rats. J

Vasc Surg. 2007 Aug;46(2):346-53. Epub 2007 Jun 27.

[30] Chancer V, Chopra, K. Role of nitric oxide in resveratrol-induced renal protective effects of ischemic preconditioning. J Vasc Surg. 2005 Dec;42(6):1198-205.

[31] Hascalik S, Celik O, et al. Resveratrol, a red wine constituent polyphenol, protects from ischemia-reperfusion damage of the ovaries. Gynecol Obstet Invest. 2004;57(4):218-23. Epub 2004 Feb 11.

[32] Karabulut AB, Kirimlioglu V, et al. Protective effects of resveratrol on spleen and ileum in rats subjectetd to ischemia-reperfusion. Transplant Proc. 2006 Mar;38(2):375-7.

[33] Hao HD, He LR. Mechanisms of cardiovascular protection by resveratrol. J Med Food. 2004 Fall;7(3):290-8.

[34] Stef G, Csiszar A, et al. Resveratrol inhibits aggregation of platelets from high-risk cardiac patients with aspirin resistance. J Cardiovasc Pharmacol. 2006 Aug;48(2):1-5.

[35] Olas B, Wachowicz B. Resveratrol, a phenolic antioxidant with effects on blood platelet functions. Platelets. 2005 Aug;16(5):251-60.

[36] Cass H. Resveratrol fights brain plaque. Nov 1, 2005. Available from: http://www.life-enhancement.com/article_template.asp?ID =1139.

[37] Marambaud P, Zhao H, et al. Resveratrol promotes clearance of Alzheimer's disease amyloid-beta peptides. J Biol Chem. 2005 Nov 11;280(45):37377-82. Epub 2005 Sep 14.

[38] Chen J, Zhou Y, et al. SIRT1 protects against microglia-dependent amyloid-beta toxicity through inhibiting NF-kappaB signaling. J Biol Chem. 2005 Dec 2;280(48):40364-74. Epub 2005 Sep 23.

[39] The French paradox for the brain. The Harvard Mahoney Neuroscience Institute Letter. On the Brain. 2007 Winter;13(1). Available from: http://www.med.harvard.edu/publications/ On_The_Brain/Volume13/OTB_Winter_07.pdf.

[40] Sukel K. Ingredients may affect brain health. Dana Foundation. Brain Work. 2007 Jul 1. Available from: http://www.dana.org/news/brainwork/detail.aspx?id=8342.

[41] Dasgupta B, Milbrandt J. Resveratrol stimulates AMP kinase activity in neurons. Proc Natl Acad Sci U S A. 2007 Apr 24;104(17):7217-22. Epub 2007 Apr 16.

[42] Lu KT, Chiou RY, et al. Neuroprotective effects of resveratrol on cerebral ischemia-induced neuron loss mediated by free radical scavenging and cerebral blood flow elevation. J Agric Food Chem. 2006 Apr 19;54(8):3126-31.

[43] Delmas D, Jannin B, et al. Resveratrol: preventing properties against vascular alterations and ageing. Mol Nutr Food Res. 2005 May;49(5):377-95.

[44] Ates O, Cayli S, et al. Neuroprotection by resveratrol against traumatic brain injury in rats. Mol Cell Biochem. 2007 Jan;294(1-2):137-44. Epub 2006 Aug 19.

[45] Robb SJ, Robb-Gaspers LD, et al. Influence of calcium and iron on cell death and mitochondrial function in oxidatively stressed astrocytes.. J Neurosci Res. 1999 Mar 15;55(6):674-86.

[46] Mokni M, Aouani E, et al. Effect of resveratrol on antioxidant enzymes in the brain of healthy rats. Neurochem Res. 2007 Jun;32(6):981-7.

[47] Zhuang H, Kim YS, et al. Potential mechanism by which resveratrol, a red wine constituent, protects neurons. Ann N Y Acad Sci. 2003 May;993:276-86; discussion 287-8.

[48] Doré S. Unique properties of polyphenol stilbenes in the brain: more than direct antioxidant actions, gene/protein regulatory activity. Neurosignals. 2005;14(1-2):61-70.

[49] Borten O, Liberman A, et al. Effects of dietary restriction and metal supplementation on the accumulation of iron-laden glial inclusions in the aging rat hippocampus. Biogerontology. 2004;5(2):81-8.

[50] National Cancer Institute [homepage on the Internet]. Executive Summary of Inflammation and Cancer Think Tank. Available from: http://www.cancer.gov/think-tanks-cancer-biology/page8.

[51] La Casa C, de la Lastra CA, et al. Resveratrol, a polyphenol found in grapes, suppresses oxidative damage and stimulates apoptosis during early colonic inflammation in rats. Biochem Pharmacol. 2004 Apr 1;67(7):1399-410.

[52] Jang M, Cai L, et al. Cancer chemopreventive activity of resveratrol, a natural product derived from grapes. Science. 1997 Jan 10;275(5297):218-20.

[53] Baur JA, Sinclair DA. Therapeutic potential of resveratrol: the in vivo evidence. Nat Rev Drug Discov. 2006 Jun;5(6):493-506. Epub 2006 May 26.

[54] Aggarwal BB, Shishodia S, editors. Resveratrol in health and disease. Boca Raton (FL): Taylor & Francis Group; 2006.

[55] Anderson J, et al. Lifestyle or resveratrol? Comparison of white and red wine consumption and colorectal neoplasia. Proceedings from the 2006 annual meeting of the American College of Gastroenterology. Las Vegas, NV. Abstract #920. 2006 Oct 23-25.

[56] Webb PM, Purdie DM, et al. Alcohol, wine, and risk of epithelial ovarian cancer. Cancer Epidemiol Biomarkers Prev. 2004 Apr;13(4):592-9.

[57] Briggs NC, Levine RS, et al. Wine drinking and risk of non-Hodgkin's lymphoma among men in the United States: a population-based case-control study. Am J Epidemiol. 2002 Sep 1;156(5):454-62.

[58] Schoonen WM, Salinas CA, et al. Alcohol consumption and risk of prostate cancer in middle-aged men. Int J Cancer. 2005 Jan 1;113(1):133-40.

[59] Potter GA, Patterson LH, et al. The cancer preventative agent resveratrol is converted to the anticancer agent piceatannol by the

cytochrome P450 enzyme CYP1B1. Br J Cancer. 2002 Mar 4;86(5):774-8.

[60] Barstad B, Sørensen TI, et al. Intake of wine, beer and spirits and risk of gastric cancer. Eur J Cancer Prev. 2005 Jun;14(3):239-43.

[61] Lappe JM, Travers-Gustafson D, et al. Vitamin D and calcium supplementation reduces cancer risk: results of a randomized trial. Am J Clin Nutr. 2007 Jun;85(6):1586-91.

[62] Wright M, Albanes D, et al. Development of a comprehensive dietary antioxidant index and application to lung cancer risk in a cohort of male smokers. Am J Epidemiol. 2004 Jul 1;160(1):68-76.

[63] Block JB, Evans S. Clinical evidence supporting cancer risk reduction with antioxidants and implications for diet and supplementation. J Am Nutra Assoc. 2000 Fall;3(3):6-16.

[64] Ames BN. DNA damage from micronutrient deficiencies is likely to be a major cause of cancer. Metat Res. 2001 Apr 18;475(1-2):7-20.

[65] Lambert JD, Hong J, et al. Inhibition of carcinogenesis by polyphenols: evidence from laboratory investigations. Am J Clin Nutr. 2005;81(1 Suppl):284S-291S.

[66] Williams MT, Hord NG. The role of dietary factors in cancer prevention: beyond fruits and vegetables. Nutr Clin Pract. 2005 Aug;20(4):451-9.

[67] Aggarwal BB, Shishodia S, editors. Resveratrol in health and disease. Boca Raton (FL): Taylor & Francis Group; 2006.

[68] Lappe JM, Travers-Gustafson D, et al. Vitamin D and calcium supplementation reduces cancer risk: results of a randomized trial. Am J Clin Nutr. 2007 Jun;85(6):1586-91.

[69] Hong WK, Sporn MB. Recent advances in chemoprevention of cancer. Science. 1997 Nov 7;278(5340):1073-7.

[70] Jemal A, Siegel R, et al. Cancer statistics, 2007. CA Cancer J Clin. 2007 Jan-Feb;57(1):43-66.

[71] Jang M, Cai L, et al. Cancer chemopreventive activity of resveratrol,

a natural product derived from grapes. Science. 1997 Jan 10;275(5297):218-20.

[72] Pezzuto JM. Resveratrol as an inhibitor of carcinogenesis. In: Aggarwal BB, Shishodia S, editors. Resveratrol in health and disease. Boca Raton (FL): Taylor & Francis Group; 2006.

[73] Pezzuto JM. Resveratrol as an inhibitor of carcinogenesis. In: Aggarwal BB, Shishodia S, editors. Resveratrol in health and disease. Boca Raton (FL): Taylor & Francis Group; 2006.

[74] Pezzuto JM. Resveratrol as an inhibitor of carcinogenesis. In: Aggarwal BB, Shishodia S, editors. Resveratrol in health and disease. Boca Raton (FL): Taylor & Francis Group; 2006.

[75] Aziz MH, Kumar R, et al. Cancer chemoprevention by resveratrol: in vitro and in vivo studies and the underlying mechanisms (review). Intl J Oncol. 2003 Jul;23(1):17-28.

[76] Aggarwal BB, Shishodia S, editors. Resveratrol in health and disease. Boca Raton (FL): Taylor & Francis Group; 2006.

[77] Docherty JJ, Fu MM, et al. Effect of resveratrol on herpes simplex virus vaginal infection in the mouse. Antiviral Res. 2005 Sep;67(3):155-62.

[78] Su JL, Yang CY, et al. Forkhead proteins are critical for bone morphogenetic protein-2 regulation and anti-tumor activity of resveratrol. J Biol Chem. 2007 Jul 6;282(27):19385-98. Epub 2007 May 18.

[79] Potter GA, Patterson LH, et al. The cancer preventative agent resveratrol is converted to the anticancer agent piceatannol by the cytochrome P450 enzyme CYP1B1. Br J Cancer. 2002 Mar 4;86(5):774-8.

[80] Kaldas MI, Walle UK, et al. Resveratrol transport and metabolism by human intestinal Caco-2 cells. J Pharm Pharmacol. 2003 Mar;55(3):307-12.

[81] Gescher AJ, Steward WP. Relationship between mechanisms, bioavailibility, and preclinical chemopreventive efficacy of resveratrol:

a conundrum. Cancer Epidemiol Biomarkers Prev. 2003 Oct;12(10):953-7.

[82] Leiro J, Orallo F, et al. Effect of cis-resveratrol on genes involved in nuclear factor kappa B signaling. Int Immunopharmacol. 2005 Feb:5(2):393-406.

[83] Leiro J, Orallo F, et al. Effects of cis-resveratrol on inflammatory murine macrophages: antioxidant activity and down-regulation of inflammatory genes. J Leukoc Biol. 2004 Jun;75(6):1156-65. Epub 2004 Feb 24.

[84] Prokop J, Sovak M, et al. Resveratrol and its glycon piceid are stable polyphenols. J Med Food. 2006 Spring;9(1):11-4.

[85] Prokop J, Sovak M, et al. Resveratrol and its glycon piceid are stable polyphenols. J Med Food. 2006 Spring;9(1):11-4.

[86] Baur JA, Sinclair DA. Therapeutic potential of resveratrol: the in vivo evidence. Nat Rev Drug Discov. 2006 Jun;5(6):493-506. Epub 2006 May 26.

Chapter 7

[1] Scalbert A, Manach C, et al. Dietary polyphenols and the prevention of diseases. Crit Rev Food Sci Nutr. 2005;45(4):287-306.

[2] Lotito SB, Frei B. Consumption of flavonoid-rich foods and increased plasma antioxidant capacity in humans: cause, consequence, or epiphenomenon? Free Radic Biol Med. 2006 Dec 15;41(12):1727-46. Epub 2006 Jun 3.

[3] Vita JA. Polyphenols and cardiovascular disease: effects on endothelial and platelet function. Am J Clin Nutr. 2005 Jan;81(1 Suppl):292S-297S.

[4] Lotito SB, Frei B. Consumption of flavonoid-rich foods and

increased plasma antioxidant capacity in humans: cause, consequence, or epiphenomenon? Free Radic Biol Med. 2006 Dec 15;41(12):1727-46. Epub 2006 Jun 3.

[5] Scalbert A, Johnson IT, et al. Polyphenols: antioxidants and beyond. Am J Clin Nutr. 2005 Jan;81(1 Suppl):215S-217S.

[6] Scalbert A, Johnson IT, et al Polyphenols: antioxidants and beyond. Am J Clin Nutr. 2005 Jan;81(1 Suppl):215S-217S.

[7] Ignarro LJ. NO more heart disease. 1st ed. New York: St. Martin's Press; 2005.

[8] Carreras MC, Schöpfer F, et al. Mitochondrial function and nitric oxide utilization. Biol Res. 2000;33(2):177-83.

[9] Nisoli E, Clementi E, et al. Mitochondrial biogenesis in mammals: the role of endogenous nitric oxide. Science. 2003 Feb 7;299(5608):896-9.

[10] Ignarro LJ. NO more heart disease. 1st ed. New York: St. Martin's Press; 2005.

[11] Stuart-Smith K. Demystified. Nitric oxide. Mol Pathol. 2002 Dec;55(6):360-6.

[12] Ignarro LJ. NO more heart disease. 1st ed. New York: St. Martin's Press; 2005.

[13] Leikert JF, Räthel TR, et al. Red wine polyphenols enhance endothelial nitric oxide synthase expression and subsequent nitric oxide release from endothelial cells. Circulation. 2002 Sep 24;106(13):1614-7.

[14] Bernátová I, Pechánová O, et al. Wine polyphenols improve cardiovascular remodeling and vascular function in NO-deficient hypertension. Am J Physiol Heart Circ Physiol. 2002 Mar;282(3):H942-8.

[15] Curin Y, Ritz MF, et al. Cellular mechanisms of the protective effect of polyphenols on the neurovascular unit in strokes. Cardiovasc Hematol Agents Med Chem. 2006 Oct;4(4):277-88.

[16] Leighton F, Miranda-Rottmann S, et al. A central role of eNOS in the protective effect of wine against metabolic syndrome. Cell Biochem Funct. 2006 Jul-Aug;24(4):291-8.

[17] Leikert JF, Räthel TR, et al. Red wine polyphenols enhance endothelial nitric oxide synthase expression and subsequent nitric oxide release from endothelial cells. Circulation. 2002 Sep 24;106(13):1614-7.

[18] Bernal-Mizracki C, Bates AC, et al. Vascular respiratory uncoupling increases blood pressure and atherosclerosis. Nature. 2005 May 26;435(7041):502-6.

[19] Ignarro LJ. NO more heart disease. 1st ed. New York: St. Martin's Press; 2005.

[20] Stein JH, Keevil JG, et al. Purple grape juice improves endothelial function and reduces the susceptibility of LDL cholesterol to oxidation in patients with coronary artery disease. Circulation. 1999 Sep 7;100(10):1050-5.

[21] Knekt P, Kumpulainen J, et al. Flavonoid intake and risk of chronic diseases. Am J Clin Nutr. 2002 Sep;76(3):560-8.

[22] Knekt P, Kumpulainen J, et al. Flavonoid intake and risk of chronic diseases. Am J Clin Nutr. 2002 Sep;76(3):560-8.

[23] Lekakis J, Rallidis LS, et al. Polyphenolic compounds from red grapes acutely improve endothelial function in patients with coronary heart disease. Eur J Cardiovasc Prev Rehabil. 2005 Dec;12(6):596-600.

[24] Castilla P, Echarri R, et al. Concentrated red grape juice exerts antioxidant, hypolipidemic, and antiinflammatory effects in both hemodialysis patients and healthy subjects. Am J Clin Nutr. 2006 Jul;84(1):252-62.

[25] Zern TL, Wood RJ, et al. Grape polyphenols exert a cardioprotective effect in pre- and postmenopausal women by lowering plasma lipids and reducing oxidative stress. J Nutr. 2005 Aug;135(8):1911-7.

[26] Choi YJ, Kang JS, et al. Polyphenolic flavonoids differ in their antiapoptotic efficacy in hydrogen peroxide-treated human vascular endothelial cells. J Nutr. 2003 Apr;133(4):985-91.

[27] Frank J. Beyond vitamin E supplementation; an alternative strategy to improve vitamin E status. J Plant Physiol. 2005 Jul;162(7):834-43.

[28] Peres W, Tuñón MJ, et al. The flavonoid quercetin ameliorates liver damage in rats with biliary obstruction. J Hepatol. 2000 Nov;33(5):742-50.

[29] Hubbard GP, Wolffram S, et al. Ingestion of onion soup high in quercetin inhibits platelet aggregation and essential components of the collagen-stimulated platelet activation pathway in man: a pilot study. Br J Nutr. 2006 Sep;96(3):482-8.

[30] Lakhanpal P, Rai DK. Quercetin: a versatile flavonoid. Internet J of Med Update. 2007 Jul-Dec;2(2): http://www.geocities.com/agnihotrimed/paper05_jul-dec2007.htm.

[31] Corder R, Mullen W, er al. Oenology: red wine procyanidins and vascular health. Nature. 2006 Nov 30;444(7119):566.

[32] Natella F, Belelli F, et al. Grape seed proanthocyanidins prevent plasma postprandial oxidative stress in humans. J Agric Food Chem. 2002 Dec 18;50(26):7720-5.

[33] Katiyar SK. Dietary grape seed proanthocyanidins inhibit photocarcinogenesis through prevention of UV-induced suppression of immune responses via induction of interleukin-12 in mice. Presented at the 233rd national meeting of the American Chemical Society, Chicago, March 25, 2007. Abstract: AGFD 011.

[34] Hughes-Formella B, Wunderlich O, et al. Anti-inflammatory and skin-hydrating properties of a dietary supplement and topical formulations containing oligomeric proanthocyanidins. Skin Pharmacol Physiol. 2007;20(1):43-9. Epub 2006 Oct 11.

[35] Kaur M, Agarwal C, et al. Grape seed extract inhibits in vitro and in vivo growth of human colorectal carcinoma cells. Clin Cancer Res. 2006 Oct 15;12(20 Pt 1):6194-202.

[36] Oligomeric proanthocyanidins (OPCs). Monograph. Alt Med Rev. 2003 Nov;8(4):442-50.

[37] Sterling M. Got anthocyanins? Nutrition Science News. 2001 Dec. Available from: http://www.newhope.com/nutritionsciencenews/nsn_backs/Dec_01/antho.cfm.

Chapter 8

[1] Perricone N. The perricone prescription. Paperback ed. New York: HarperResource; 2004.

[2] Hughes-Formela B, Wunderlich O, et al. Anti-inflammatory and skin-hydrating properties of a dietary supplement and topical formulations containing oligomeric proanthocyanidins. Skin Pharmacol Physiol. 2007;20(1):43-9. Epub 2006 Oct 11.

[3] Heinrich U, Stahl W. Long-term ingestion of high flavanol cocoa provides photoprotection against UV-induced erythema and improves skin condition in women. J Nutr. 2006 Jun;136(6):1565-9.

[4] Heinrich U, Tronnier H, et al. Antioxidant supplements improve parameters related to skin structure in humans. Skin Pharmacol Physiol. 2006;19(4):224-31.

[5] Sunburn prevalence among adults—United States, 1999, 2003, and 2004. MMWR. 2007;56(21):524-528. Centers for Disease Control and Prevention (CDC).

[6] Aziz MH, Reagan-Shaw S, et al. Chemoprevention of skin cancer by grape constituent resveratrol: relevance to human disease? FASEB J. 2005 Jul;19(9):1193-5. Epub 2005 Apr 18.

[7] Aggarwal BB, Bhardwai A, et al. Role of resveratrol in prevention and therapy of cancer: preclinical and clinical studies. Anticancer Res. 2004 Sep-Oct;24(5A):2783-840.

[8] Martin KR. Targeting apoptosis with dietary bioactive agents. Exp Biol Med (Maywood). 2006 Feb;231(2):117-29.

[9] Sies H, Stahl W. Nutritional protection against skin damage from sunlight. Annu Rev Nutr. 2004;24:173-200.

[10] Perricone N. The perricone prescription. Paperback ed. New York: HarperResource; 2004.

[11] Mittal A, Elmets CA, et al. Dietary feeding of proanthocyanidins from grape seeds prevents photocarcinogenesis in SKH-1 hairless mice: relationship to decreased fat and lipid peroxidation. Carcinogenesis. 2003 Aug;24(8):1379-88. Epub 2003 Jun 5.

[12] Han B. Nimni M. Proanthocyanidin: a natural crosslinking reagent for stabilizing collagen matrices. J Biomed Mater Res A. 2003 Apr 1;65(1):118-24.

[13] Oligomeric proanthocyanidins (OPCs). Monograph. Alt Med Rev. 2003 Nov;8(4):442-50.

[14] Maffei Facino R, Carini M, et al. Free radical scavenging action and anti-enzyme activities of procyanidines from vitis vinifera. A mechanism for their capillary protective action. Arzneimittelforschung. 1994 May;44(5):592–601.

[15] Frank J, Budek A, et al. Dietary flavonoids with a catechol structure increase alpha-tocopherol in rats and protect the vitamin from oxidation in vitro. J Lipid Res. 2006 Dec;47(12):2718-25. Epub 2006 Sep 1.

[16] Peres W, Tuñón MJ, et al. The flavonoid quercetin ameliorates liver damage in rats with biliary obstruction. J Hepatol. 2000 Nov;33(5):742-50.

[17] Arck PD, Peters EM, et al. Towards a "free radical theory of graying:" melanocyte apoptosis in the aging human hair follicle is an indicator of oxidative stress induced tissue damage. FASEB J. 2006 Jul;20(9):1567-9. Epub 2006 May 24.

[18] Takahasi T, Kamiya T, et al. Procyanidin oligomers selectively and intensively promote proliferation of mouse hair epithelial cells in vitro and activate hair follicle growth in vivo. J Invest Dermatol. 1999 Mar;112(3):310-6.

[19] Fujita S, Volpi E. Amino acids and muscle loss with aging. J Nutr. 2006 Jan;136(1 Suppl):277S-89S.

[20] Herbst A, Pak JW, et al. Accumulation of mitochondrial DNA deletion mutations in aged muscle fibers: evidence for a causal role in muscle fiber loss. J Gerontol A Biol Sci Med Sci. 2007 Mar;62(3):235-45.

[21] Semba RD, Blaum C, et al. Carotenoid and vitamin E status are associated with indicators of sarcopenia among older women living in the community. Aging Clin Exp Res. 2003 Dec;15(6):482-7.

[22] Stephens FB, Constantin-Teodosiu D, et al. New insights concerning the role of carnitine in the regulation of fuel metabolism in skeletal muscle. J Physiol. 2007 Jun 1;581(Pt 2):431-44. Epub 2007 Mar 1.

Chapter 9

[1] Ames BN, Atamna H, et al. Mineral and vitamin deficiencies can accelerate the mitochondrial decay of aging. Mol Aspects Med. 2005 Aug-Oct;26(4-5):363-78.

[2] Davis DR, Epp MD, et al. Changes in USDA food composition data for 43 garden crops, 1950 to 1999. J Am Coll Nutr. 2004 Dec;23(6):669-82.

[3] Ames BN. Low micronutrient intake may accelerate the degenerative diseases of aging through allocation of scarce micronutrients by triage. Proc Natl Acad Sci U S A. 2006 Nov 21;103(47):17589-94. Epub 2006 Nov 13.

[4] Lau FC, Shukitt-Hale B, et al. Nutritional intervention in brain aging: reducing the effects of inflammation and stress. Subcell Biochem. 2007;42:299-318.

[5] Liu RH. Health benefits of fruit and vegetables are from additive and synergistic combinations of phytochemicals. Am J Clin Nutr. 2003 Sep;78(3 Suppl):517S-520S.

INDEX

hair changes, 131-132
and UV radiation, 126-127
sleep deprivation, and
inflammation/oxidation, 37
smoking
and antioxidant use, 95
and French Paradox, 3
and inflammation, 25, 33
as risk factor in disease, 19
spinal cord, and acetyl L-carnitine,
69
spleen, and resveratrol, 85
statin therapy, for high cholesterol,
30-31
stress
and inflammation, 25, 34
as risk factor in disease, 19
stroke
See also heart disease
acetyl L-carnitine and, 69
alpha lipoic acid and, 65-66, 146
nitric oxide and, 85, 112
resveratrol and, 91, 93, 143
sugar
and inflammation, 25, 36
as risk factor in disease, 19
Sumpio, Bauer, on red wine
polyphenols, 17
superoxide dismutase (SOD),
antioxidant enzyme, 25
supplementation, reasons for,
136-138
synergy *See* polyphenols, synergy
of

T
Thun, Michael, on Harvard study,
11
trans fats
and cholesterol, 36

heart disease and, 12-13, 18
and inflammation, 25, 36
as risk factor in disease, 19
and skin damage, 125
triglycerides, and adipose tissue, 68
tumors *See* cancer
Type 2 diabetes *See* insulin
resistance

U
ubiquinol *See* coenzyme Q-10
Universal Antioxidant *See* alpha
lipoic acid
uric acid, antioxidant, 26
UV radiation, and skin, 126-127

V
vegetables
See also whole foods
and inflammation, 34-35
vitamin C *See* mitochondrial
antioxidants
vitamin D, and cancer, 95-96
vitamin E
See also mitochondrial
antioxidants
and muscle, 133-134
and quercetin, 117
vitamin supplements
See also supplementation
for mitochondrial support,
60-61

W
Weil, Andrew, on inflammation, 23
white blood cells, in inflammation,
24, 29
whole foods, 138-139
wine consumption, 3, 5-6, 17
wrinkles *See* skin health

Renaissance Health Education, LLC
925 S. Federal Highway, Suite 500
Boca Raton, Florida 33432
www.naturalhealthnewsreport.com